Biostatistics in <u>*Health Research*</u>

Third Edition

Dr Uttam Kumar Roy MBBS, DCH, MD
Professor
Department of Pharmacology and Therapeutics
Burdwan Medical College & Hospital
(West Bengal, India)

Dr. Shouvik Choudhury MBBS, MD
Assistant Professor
Department of Pharmacology and Therapeutics
Burdwan Medical College & Hospital
(West Bengal, India)

Foreword

It is my pleasure to write the Foreword of the book "Biostatistics in Health Research" by Dr. Uttam Kumar Roy, Associate professor of Pharmacology and Therapeutics at Burdwan Medical College and Hospital. Research is the cornerstone of medical education and high-quality health care. One of the NIH quotes wrote "Institutes with a tradition of excellence have amply demonstrated that research enhances the vitality of teaching, teaching lifts the standards of care, and patient care opens up new avenues of investigation."

However, one of the reasons for not having many clinician scientists in our country is lack of research culture and training. Even a superficial look at the content of this book is enough to realize that this book is an attempt to bridge the gap of inadequate research training among undergraduate and postgraduate students in the country. The unique features of the book include competency-based lessons, attempt towards skill development through solved problems, avoidance of much mathematics to which medical students are less versed, learning data analysis even without software based largely on tables, and figures. The author is a dedicated teacher. I believe that this book will be an asset for research training among undergraduate and postgraduate students and clinician scientists not only within India but also elsewhere.

Uday C Ghoshal

Professor and Head

Department of Gastroenterology

Sanjay Gandhi Postgraduate Institute of Medical Sciences

Lucknow, India

Email: udayghoshal@gmail.com

Preface to First Edition

"Biostatistics in Health Research" has been written for those who are engaged in research activities in medical and allied health sciences. Readers will require only basic knowledge in mathematics or statistics. Author has focused on those points which readers must know and have been presented with numerous tables, flow charts and images for better understanding of the subject matter related to biomedical research. Main characteristic feature of this book is that it is competency based, skill development through examples and any one can learn the topic in a very short period of time. For the beginners, it is easy to proceed through excel without need for a software. Wherever possible, little text materials have been added. Most of the statistical tests are followed by examples and solved with the help of excel to develop skill in calculation through stepwise approach. Frequently asked questions are other aspect of the book where I have touched any basic knowledge about a topic which is not included in the text. Also, for assessment of other discussed topic, few questions have been provided to revise and test your knowledge. Terms related to interventional study will simplify the complicated portion of trial process. Overall readers will learn biostatistics in a very short time without need of a software. I started writing from my postgraduate trainee period, revised again and again and updated periodically. Finally, my co-author Dr Shouvik Choudhury helped me very much and gave it a final shape. No book is flawless and we would really appreciate your constructive criticism (uroy951@gmail.com). Dr Uttam Kumar Roy (MBBS.DCH.MD)

Acknowledgement

First of all, we express our heartfelt acknowledgement to Prof (Dr) Abhijit Das, Head of the Department, Department of Pharmacology, Burdwan Medical College & Hospital (WB) for his constant encouragement. We shall remain ever grateful to Dr (Prof) Santanu Kumar Tripathi, Principal, Netaji Subhas Medical College & Hospital, Bihta (Patna, India) who inspired us all throughout the journey in writing this book.

Authors are deeply indebted to the following doctors for their constant support:

Prof (Dr) Pinaki Chakravarty, Head of the Department of Pharmacology, Tezpur Medical College (Assam)

Prof. (Dr.) Suparna Chatterjee, Professor of Pharmacology, IPGME&R Kolkata

Prof. (Dr.) Avijit Hazra, Professor of Pharmacology, IPGME&R Kolkata

Dr Diptimoyee Devi (Professor & Head of the department of Pharmacology& Therapeutics, Gauhati Medical College (Assam, India)

Dr Rahul Ghosh Hazra, Assistant prof. of Pharmacology, Burdwan Medical College & Hospital (WB)

Dr Somiran Malakar, Dr. Zishan Akhtar, Dr Nazibul Haque (MD PGT), Burdwan Medical College & Hospital (WB)

Dr Uttam Kumar Roy

Dr Shouvik Choudhury

Abbreviations

ANCOVA	Analysis of Covariance
ANOVA	Analysis of Variance
CFR	Case Fatality Rate
CI	Confidence Interval
CV	Coefficient of Variation
CVI	Content Validity Index
DF	Degree of Freedom
DV	Dependent Variable
FGD	Focus Group Discussion
FINER	Feasible, Interesting, Novel, Ethical, Relevant
GCP	Good Clinical Practice
IND	Investigational New Drug
IQR	Inter Quartile Range
IV	Independent Variable
KM plot	Kaplan-Meier Plot
MANOVA	Multivariate Analysis of Variance
MH Test	Mantel-Hanszel test
MLE	Maximum Likelihood Estimation
NNH	Number Needed to Harm
NNT	Number Needed to Treat
NPV	Negative Predictive Value
OFAT	One Factor at a Time
OLS	Ordinary Least Square
OR	Odds Ratio
PPS	Probability Proportional to Size
PPV	Positive Predictive Value
PROSPERO	Prospective Register of Systematic Review
RCT	Randomized Controlled Trial
ROC	Receiver Operating Characteristic curve
RR	Relative Risk
SD	Standard Deviation
SEM	Standard Error of Mean
SMART	Specific, Measurable, Achievable, Relevant, Time
SPANOVA	Split Plot ANOVA
SPSS	Statistical Packages for Social Sciences
SRS	Simple Random Sampling
SS	Sum of Squares

Table of Contents

Chapter 1: Introduction *1*
    Section 1: Basic Terms Used in Statistics 1
    Section 2: Mathematics in Biology 2

Chapter 2: Basics of Biostatistics *4*
    Section 1: Types of Data 4
    Section 2: Scales of Measurement of Data 5
    Section 3: Measure of Central Tendency 6
    Section 4: Measures of Dispersion of Data 7
    Section 5: Presentation of Data 14
    Section 6: Distribution of Data 21
    Section 7: Data Transformation 25

Chapter 3: Hypothesis Testing *26*
    Section 1: Hypothesis Testing 26
    Section 2: Terms Related to Hypothesis Testing 28
    Section 3: Frequently Asked Questions 37

Chapter 4: Types of Study *38*
    Section 1: Different Types of Study 38
    Section 2: Important terms 49
    Section 3: Conducting Different Types of Study 54
    Section 4: Confounding in Research 56

Chapter 5: Measures of Health Outcome *58*
    Section 1: Measures of Disease Frequency 58
    Section 2: Frequently Asked Questions 63

Chapter 6: Statistical Tests *65*
    Section 1: Statistical Procedure 65
    Section 2: Assumptions of Statistical Test 69
    Section 3: Student t Test 73

Table of Contents

Section 4: Analysis of Variance (ANOVA) 82
Section 5: Chi-Square Test 109
Section 6: Non-parametric Test 116

Chapter 7: Study Design 119
Section 1: Common Types of Study Design 119
Section 2: FAQ on Study Design 125

Chapter 8: Correlation and Regression 126
Section 1: Correlation 126
Section 2: Regression Analysis 129

Chapter 9: Bias in Medical Research 140
Section 1: Bias 140
Section 2: Statistical Errors (Flow Chart) 143

Chapter 10: Evaluation of a Test or Tool 144
Section 1: Validity and Reliability 144
Section 2: Frequently Asked Questions 147

Chapter 11: Diagnostic Test Study 149
Section 1: Validity for Binary Data 149
Section 2: Validity for Continuous Data 152

Chapter 12: Measures of Agreement 154
Section 1: Understanding Agreement 154
Section 2: Common Measures of Agreement 155

Chapter 13: Survival Analysis 158
Section 1: Basic Understanding of Survival Analysis 158
Section 2: Frequently Asked Questions 160

Chapter 14: Sampling 161
Section 1: Different Terms Used in Sampling 161
Section 2: Sampling Technique 163

Table of Contents

Chapter 15: Sample Size Calculation...................................170

   Section 1: Concept behind Sample Size Calculation 170

   Section 2: Sample Size Calculation 171

Chapter 16: Systematic Review..176

   Section 1: Systematic Review and Metanalysis 176

   Section 2: FAQ on Systematic Review 179

   Section 3: Systematic Review Process (Flow Chart)......................181

Chapter 17: Assessments 182

   Section 1: Type of Study 182

   Section 2: Type of Analysis...185

Bibliography 187

INDEX...190

Chapter 1: Introduction

Section 1: Basic Terms Used in Statistics

Statistics

Science and art of handling aggregates of information-observation, enumeration, recording, classifying and systematically treating them. If information collected is related with biological sciences, it is known as Biostatistics.

Population & Sample

All individuals or objects of specific characteristic in a defined area. It may be finite when total number can be counted, or it may be infinite. Sample is a finite number of units selected from the population. So, it is part of the population.

Variable

A characteristic feature of individuals in a population (or a sample) which varies from one individual to another and/or, for the same individual, from one point of time to another. Examples include Height, Weight, BP, Reaction time, Gender etc.

Data

An organized collection of information, containing values of the variables. Systolic BP (Variable) recorded 120 mm Hg (Data).

Parameter & Statistic

Parameter represents measures of population whereas Statistic represents measures of sample. By convention, Statistic is denoted by Roman letters and the parameters by Greek letters (Sample mean by $\bar{X}$ and Population mean by μ)

Model

Relationship between two or more variables expressed in the form of an equation. Body weight (Kg) of an infant expressed in relation with age (month) is given in the form of

Body weight (Kg) = Birth weight + $(0.5 \times Age)$. Suppose birth weight is 2 Kg, and per month increase in weight is 500 gm as per model, weight of 5 months baby is 4.5Kg.

Biostatistics in Health Research

Section 2: Mathematics in Biology

Concept of Probability

The probability represents ratio of number of events occurring to that of total events. It is expressed as decimal form or percentage form. (The term probability, possibility, likelihood -all convey same sense. It means that uncertainty is there in the occurrence of an event/outcome.

Mutually Exclusive Events

When the two events cannot occur simultaneously i.e., occurrence of one event excludes the occurrence of the other event (Pass or Fail, Cured or not cured etc.)

Independent Events

Occurrence of one event does not affect occurrence of another event.

Dependent Events

Occurrence of one event affects the occurrence of the other event.

Laws of Probability

Addition rule- for mutually exclusive events: Two events are X, Y then $P(X \text{ or } Y) = P(X) + P(Y)$ and for non-mutually exclusive events (Two events can occur simultaneously): Two events are A, B then $P(A \text{ or } B) = P(A) + P(B) - P(A \text{ and } B)$

Multiplication rule- for Independent Events: Suppose two events R, S are independent, then the probability of their joint occurrence equals to product of their individual probability and is given by $P(R \text{ and } S) = P(R) \times P(S)$

For Dependent Events: Let us take an example. Two events X and Y are dependent events. Then probability that both events occur given by $P(X) \times P(Y/X)$ or $P(Y) \times P(X/Y)$- known as conditional probability.

Problem 1: Probability that a person will develop diabetes (20%) and hypertension (30%). Assuming the two events are independent, calculate the probability that a person will develop both diabetes and hypertension. Calculate the probability that a person will develop either diabetes or hypertension or both.

First Part: $0.3 \times 0.2 = 0.06 = 6\%$ will develop both conditions.

Second Part: $0.2 + 0.3 - (0.2 \times 0.3)) = 0.44 = 44\%$.

Understanding Logarithm

In this context, we should understand the basics of Logarithm as most of the data transformation (will be discussed in Chapter 2) involves logarithmic transformation. Other areas where concept of logarithm is essential has also been focused.

Term Logarithm

We are often confused and even afraid of the term logarithm. I shall try to explain this domain which is essential for us. Let us take an example: $2^3 = 8$ and if we express in terms of logarithm, it is written as $Log_2 8 = 3$(Logarithm of 8 to the base 2 equals to 3). Here 2 is the base, 3 is exponent and 8 is the value. In general, exponential expression like $X^Y = Z$ which in terms of logarithm is written as $Log_X Z = Y$.

Types Of Logarithms

Logarithm is of two types: Common logarithm where base is 10 and is expressed as Log 10 or simply Log. Another type is Natural logarithm where base is e (Euler's constant and equals to 2.71828) and written as Ln. Examples of two types are
$Log\ 100 = 2$ and $Ln(50) = 3.912$

Application of Logarithm in Biomedical Research

- ❖ Data Transformation
- ❖ Logistic Regression
- ❖ Probit Regression
- ❖ Confidence Interval (CI) estimation of Odds Ratio (OR)

Chapter 2: Basics of Biostatistics

Section 1: Types of Data

Qualitative/ Categorical (recorded in the form of text)
Nominal-Cannot be ranked. It may be dichotomous/binary (such as cured / not cured) or polychotomous (such as Blood group)
Ordinal- Follow logical hierarchy hence can be ranked. We can also assign numbers to nominal and ordinal categories although difference among those numbers do not have numerical significance (Flow Chart 1). Socioeconomic Status, Grades of Murmur, Grades of Ascites etc. are ordered in nature.

Quantitative/ Numerical Data (recorded in number)
Continuous-Can take on any value within a given range including *fraction* (Weight, Height, Blood sugar level)
Discrete- Can take on only certain discrete values within a given range (Flow Chart 1). Number of seizure episode in last 6 month during therapy is discrete numerical.

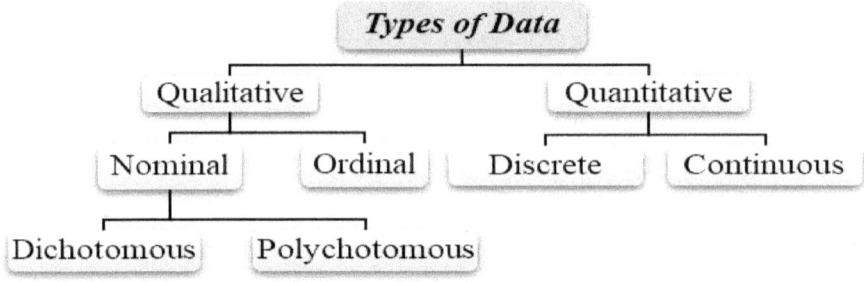

Flow Chart 1: Types of Data

Sources of Data Collection

Primary Source	Secondary Source
❖ Observation ❖ Experiment ❖ Interview ❖ Questionnaire	❖ Published source e.g. books, journal ❖ Unpublished source e.g., records in Government / private offices

Test your understanding: Sometimes Quantitative and Categorical data cannot be distinguished.

Section 2: Scales of Measurement of Data

Quantitative Scale (Flow Chart 2)
Interval Scale -Differences between two consecutive numbers carry equal significance in any part of scale unlike the scoring of an ordinal. Differences cannot be judged in the form of ratios. Here, true zero is absent. Examples include IQ, anxiety, memory etc.
Ratio Scale-It includes absolute zero. Examples include exam marks, pulse rate and income

Qualitative Scale: *Nominal scale and Ordinal scale*

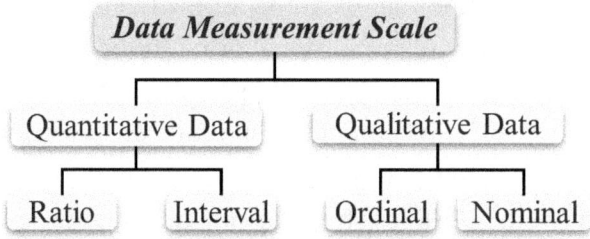

Flow Chart 2: Scale of Data Measurement

Assessment

Identify *Variables* given in Table 1 below

Table1: Health Record of Patients with Mitral Valve Disease

Subject ID	Gender	Age	Number of visits	Murmur Grades	Anemia (Grades)	Blood group
1	Male	32	2	1	Mild	A
2	Male	36	7	3	Mild	O
3	Male	38	8	5	Mild	B
4	Female	46	12	4	Severe	O
5	Female	56	6	2	Moderate	AB

Gender-Nominal Dichotomous
Age-Continuous Numerical
OPD Visits-Discrete Numerical
Grades of Murmur-Ordinal Numerical. Numbers not meaningful here, though recorded in numerical form as 5-3 ≠ 4-2
Anemia-Ordinal
Blood Groups-Nominal Polychotomous

Section 3: Measure of Central Tendency

Mean- It is of three types-arithmetic mean, geometric mean and harmonic mean (Flow Chart 3). Arithmetic mean is commonly used. Mean is of three types:

Arithmetic Mean-obtained by adding all observations divided by number of observations. This is not appropriate for qualitative data, skewed data and are sensitive to outliers.

Geometric Mean (GM)-obtained by n^{th} root of product of observations. It can handle skewed data but not applicable when data contains zero or negative values. Common applications in medicine are growth rate, % change where changes are proportional or multiplicative.

Harmonic Mean-equals Number of observations/Sum of reciprocal of observations. It is not used commonly in biomedical research.

Median- Denotes middle value (for odd number of observation) or average of two middle values (for even number of observations). Useful for data whose distribution is skewed.

Median=(n+1)/2 th term for odd number of observations
Median=Average of (n/2) th term and [(n/2) +1] th term for even number of observations

Mode-Most commonly occurring value

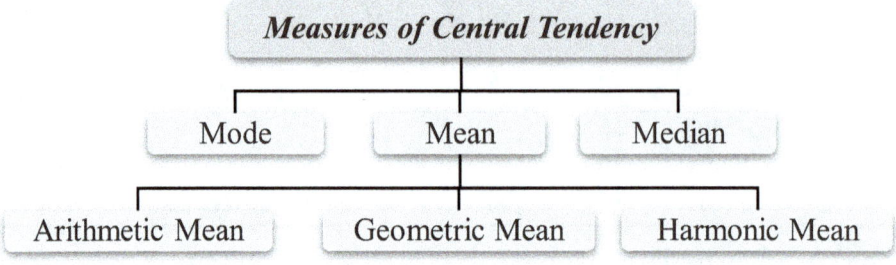

Flow Chart 3: Measures of Central Tendency

Problem 1: Reduction of viral load in four patients of hepatitis B after anti-viral drug therapy was found to be 10%, 20%, 30%, 5%. Calculate Geometric Mean (GM)

$GM = \sqrt[4]{0.1 \times 0.2 \times 0.3 \times 0.05} = 0.132$. So average reduction after therapy was 13%.

Section 4: Measures of Dispersion of Data

- ❖ Range
- ❖ Inter Quartile Range (IQR)
- ❖ Mean Deviation
- ❖ Standard Error of Mean (SEM)/Proportion
- ❖ Standard Deviation (SD) and Variance
- ❖ Coefficient of Variation (CV)

Inter Quartile Range (IQR)

When a data set has outliers or extreme values, usually it is summarized with a typical value using the median as opposed to the mean. Variability is summarized by a statistic called the IQR. The first quartile (Q1) is the value in the data set that holds 25% of the values below it. The third quartile(Q3) is the value in the data set that holds 25% of the values above it. The quartiles can be determined following the same approach that we use to determine the median, but we now consider each half of the data set separately. IQR = $Q_3 - Q_1$ (Flow Chart 4).

Even Sample Size (52,55,56,60,62,64,69,69,73,75)

For the sample as shown in Image 1 (n = 10), the median diastolic BP is 63 (50% values are above 63, and 50% are below). The quartiles can be determined in the same way we determined the median, except we consider each half of the data set separately. There are 5 values below the median (lower half), the middle value is 56 which is Q1. There are 5 values above the median (upper half), the middle value is 69 which is Q3. $IQR = 69 - 56 = 13$

Odd Sample Size (55,56,60,62,64,69,69,73,75)

When the sample size is odd (say n=9), the median and quartiles are determined in the same way (Image 2). When the sample size is 9, the median is the middle number 64. The quartiles are determined in the same way looking at the lower and upper halves, respectively. There are 4 values in the lower half, Q1 is the mean of the 2 middle values in the lower half $\frac{(56+60)}{2}$ = 58. In this way Q3= (69+73)/2=71. Then, IQR = (71 − 58 = 13).

Biostatistics in Health Research

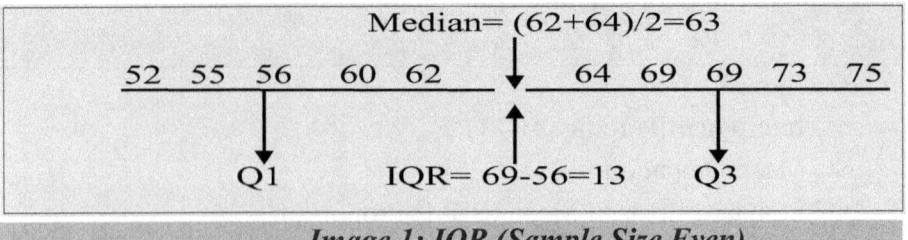

Image 1: IQR (Sample Size Even)

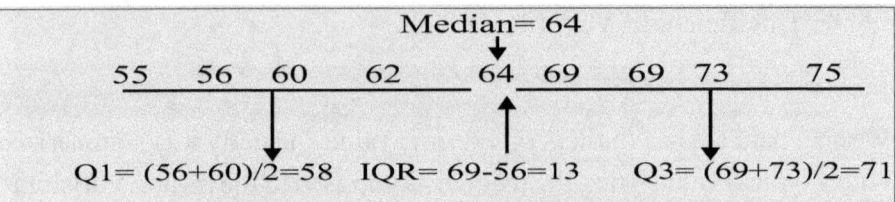

Image 2: IQR (Sample Size Odd)

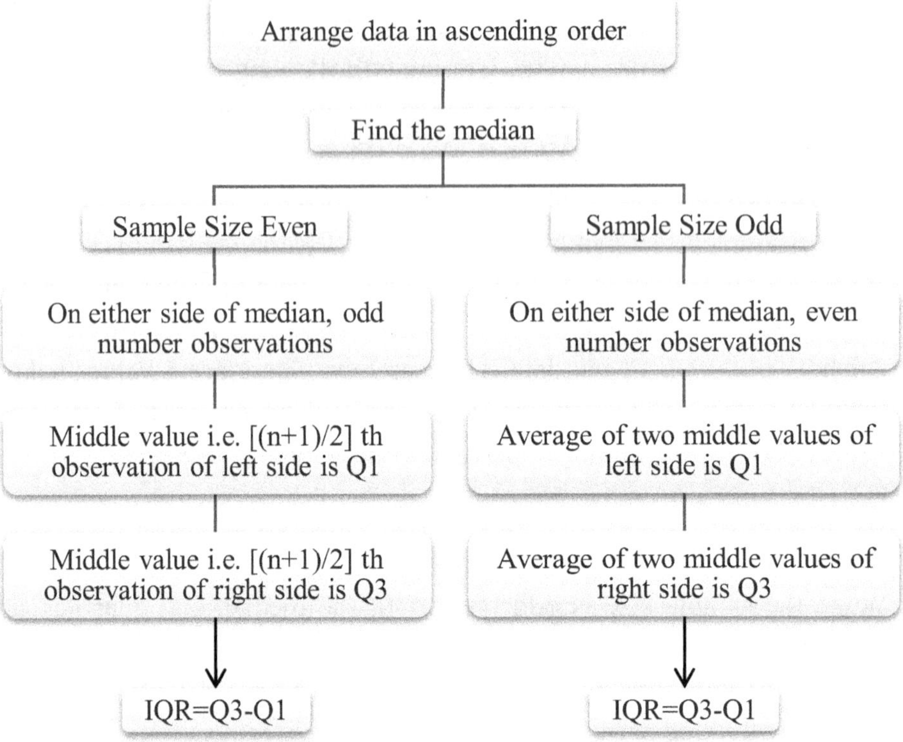

```
           Arrange data in ascending order
                        |
                  Find the median
                   /           \
        Sample Size Even     Sample Size Odd
              |                    |
   On either side of median,    On either side of median,
   odd number observations      even number observations
              |                    |
   Middle value i.e. [(n+1)/2] th   Average of two middle values of
   observation of left side is Q1   left side is Q1
              |                    |
   Middle value i.e. [(n+1)/2] th   Average of two middle values of
   observation of right side is Q3  right side is Q3
              |                    |
         IQR=Q3-Q1              IQR=Q3-Q1
```

Flow Chart 4: Steps of IQR Estimation

Standard Deviation (SD)

It is a measure of dispersion or scatter or variation of data. Other measures of dispersion are Absolute Deviation, Range, Inter Quartile Range and Variance we have more confidence while interpreting results than average value alone.

Calculation of Standard Deviation (Table 2)
Step 1: Take mean of observations
Step 2: Find difference of each value from mean
Step 3: Square the deviations
Step 4: Add all deviations
Step 5: Divide the sum by sample size in case of a sample or one less than the sample size in case of population (Variance)
Step 6: Take square root. So, $SD = \sqrt{\frac{\sum Deviation^2}{Sample\ Size}}$.

In case of sample proportion, SD is $\sqrt{pq}$ where p *is proportion with characteristic* and $q = 1 - p$.

When there are two samples where S1 and S2 are their SD, then Pooled standard deviation (Sp) is given by the formula

$Sp = \sqrt{\frac{(n_1-1)\,S_1^2 + (n_2-1)\,S_2^2}{(n_1+n_2-2)}}$

Table 2: Standard Deviation

Observation	Diff.	(Diff)²
1	4	16
2	3	9
3	2	4
6	−1	1
4	1	1
14	−9	81
Mean = 30/6 = 5		112

So, $SD(sample) = \sqrt{\frac{112}{6-1}} = \sqrt{\frac{112}{5}}$.

SD gives result in same unit and is very easy for interpretation. Variance is in squared unit and difficult to interpret. But variance have some mathematical properties which makes it useful in complex analysis. Applications of averages and measures of dispersion are displayed depending upon the types of data in Table 3 below.

Biostatistics in Health Research

Table 3: Measures of Central Tendency and Dispersion

Variable	Central tendency	Dispersion
Quantitative (no outlier)	Mean	SD
Quantitative (outlier present)	Median	IQR
Ordinal	Median	IQR
Nominal	Mode	Range

Standard Error of Mean/Proportion

In a research procedure, our idea is to draw conclusion about population parameter using sample values. If we take repeated samples of same sample size from population, we get mean for each sample and they are different from each other in most of the cases. This variability is measured by Standard Error of Mean.

Concept

If we take repeated samples from population, in each sample, we will get mean and SD. It can be shown that means of the samples will follow normal distribution. Mean of all these means of samples closely approximates population mean but sample SD is not representative of population SD. In practice, we do not collect many samples, but one large sample (observations more than 30) is taken and is supposed to be representative of population. We made a correction on SD of that sample and that is known as Standard Error of Mean (SEM) and is given by formula SEM= SD/Square Root of Sample Size ($SEM = \frac{SD}{\sqrt{n}}$). So, SD of this distribution of means of samples taken repeatedly from population is known as standard error of mean. Like SEM, we have SE of proportion, SE of difference between two means/proportions.

Standard Error of Proportion= $\sqrt{\frac{pq}{n}}$.

Thus, more the sample size, less is the SEM, and more accurate the result. That is why we always try to include as much subjects as possible.

Features of SE (Standard Error)

- ❖ SD represents variability within a sample whereas SE represents variability across samples of a population.
- ❖ Value of SD is larger than SE
- ❖ Error is less when SE is used for calculation

Application of SEM:
- Measuring variability between samples, between sample and population.
- Constructing CI for population parameter where it lies. SE is useful when drawing inference about population.

Coefficient of Variation (CV)

CV is the relative measure of dispersion of data whereas Standard Deviation represents the absolute measure. CV is expressed as the percentage of mean and is devoid of any unit making it suitable for comparing variabilities of two or more variables. SD and variance are not independent of unit. It is appropriate when variables are expressed in ratio scale as absolute zero is present here. Larger value of CV reflects less consistent and more variability compared to smaller value. $CV = \frac{SD}{Mean} *100$. It is used in two situations:

- ❖ When variables are measured in different units (Body weight and Height are two variables measured in different units. Now if we want to compare variability, CV is appropriate measure of dispersion for comparison)
- ❖ When variables are in same unit but their means vary widely (Table 4).

Table 4: Weight in Male and Female

Gender	Mean	SD
Male	60	6
Female	40	12

CV (Male) $= \frac{6}{60} \times 100$, CV (Female) $= \frac{12}{40} \times 100$, $\frac{CV(Male)}{CV(Female)} = \frac{1}{3}$

From the table, females are twice as variable as male with respect to body weight whereas CV shows females are 3 times more variable compared to male and this is to be reported in results section.

Problem 1: Systolic BP recorded in two groups (10 patients in each group). It is important to know BP of which group is more variable to avoid complications? Group1: 120, 130, 126, 134, 140, 136, 142, 148, 156, 168. Group II: 140, 158, 148, 166, 170, 172, 184, 122, 116, 110.

Basic Formulae for Beginners

- **Mean of a single proportion** $(\hat{p}) = \dfrac{Events\ of\ Interest}{Total\ Number\ of\ Trials}$

  In a trial, 40 persons out of 120 responded to therapy. Mean of proportion of response to therapy $= \dfrac{40 \times 100}{120} = 33\%\ or\ 0.33$

- **Mean of a multiple proportion** $(\bar{p}) = \dfrac{\sum_{i=1}^{k} \hat{p}_i}{k}$ where k is number of samples and $\hat{p}_i$ is sample proportion of ith sample.

  There are 4 samples and respective proportions are 0.3, 0.2, 0.1 and 0.6. Then $\bar{p} = \dfrac{0.3+0.2+0.1+0.6}{4} = 0.3$

- **Variance of a sample proportion** $= \dfrac{\hat{p}(1-\hat{p})}{n}$

  In a trial, 40 persons out of 120 responded to therapy. So, $\hat{p} = 0.33$. Using the above formula, we get variance $= \dfrac{0.33 \times (1-0.33)}{120} = 0.001843$

- **Standard deviation (SD) of a sample proportion** $= \sqrt{\dfrac{\hat{p}(1-\hat{p})}{n}}$ (Standard deviation is the square root of variance)

- Variance and SD of population proportion is given by formula $p(1-p)$ and $\sqrt{p(1-p)}$

- **Sample Variance** $= \dfrac{\sum(X_i - \bar{X})^2}{n-1}$ and **Sample SD** $= \sqrt{\dfrac{\sum(X_i - \bar{X})^2}{n-1}}$

- **Population Variance** $= \dfrac{\sum(X_i - \mu)^2}{n-1}$ and **Sample SD** $= \sqrt{\dfrac{\sum(X_i - \mu)^2}{n-1}}$

Combine Variances of Two Independent Samples

Equal sample sizes: If variances of two samples be σ_x^2 and σ_y^2, then Combined Variance $= \sigma_x^2 + \sigma_y^2$

Combined (Pooled) SD $= \sqrt{\sigma_x^2 + \sigma_y^2}$ (adding two SD to get combined SD is wrong, first get variance and then take square root. But Combined variance is obtained by simply adding two variances).

Unequal sample sizes: Now when the size of the sample varies (Suppose n_x and n_y) then Pooled Variance $= \dfrac{(n_x-1)\sigma_x^2 + (n_y-1)\sigma_y^2}{n_x + n_x - 2}$,

$$SD_{Pooled} = \sqrt{\frac{(n_x-1)\sigma_x^2+(n_y-1)\sigma_y^2}{n_x+n_x-2}}$$

If Variances of two sample proportions $\frac{p_1(1-p_1)}{n}$ and $\frac{p_2(1-p_2)}{n}$, then combined variance of two proportions $= \frac{p_1(1-p_1)}{n} + \frac{p_2(1-p_2)}{n}$. Combined SD of two proportions $= \sqrt{\frac{p_1(1-p_1)}{n} + \frac{p_2(1-p_2)}{n}}$.

When size of the sample varies (Suppose n_x and n_y) then formula for Combined Variance of two proportion $= \frac{p_1(1-p_1)}{n_x} + \frac{p_2(1-p_2)}{n_y}$ Combined SD of two proportions $= \sqrt{\frac{p_1(1-p_1)}{n_x} + \frac{p_2(1-p_2)}{n_y}}$

Combine Variances of Two Dependent Samples

All the above formulae for combined variance and SD are applicable when samples are independent. Covariance for two independent samples is zero, but if the samples are dependent then Combined variance and SD includes Covariance. This covariance adjusts for joint variability. For calculation of covariance, only paired sample size is considered but means are calculated as usual. If variances of two dependent samples be σ_x^2 and σ_y^2, then Combined Variance $= \sigma_x^2 + \sigma_y^2 + 2 \times Cov(X,Y)$. In case of dependent samples, same subjects are being used and paired measurements are taken under different treatments or different time periods. Blood pressure measurement before therapy and after therapy from same group of individual and testing variances is important. This is dependent sample. I am not going to discuss in details of calculation of covariance and combined variance for dependent samples.

Section 5: Presentation of Data

Graphical method of presentation

Qualitative data	Quantitative data
Pie chart	Frequency polygon
Bar diagram	Cumulative frequency curve
Histogram	Cumulative % frequency curve
Ogive	Box whisker plot
Population pyramid	Scatter plot
Histogram	

Ogive

This is a cumulative frequency distribution graph of grouped data. It gives us idea about how many data values lie above or below a particular value in a data set. Two types of ogives can be drawn from a sample distribution: Less Than Type (considering upper boundary) and Greater Than Type (considering lower boundary) ogive.

From a set of distribution, cumulative frequencies are calculated for each class interval (Table 5). Convert it into a continuous distribution if not. Then taking the upper-class limit in case of less than type and lower-class limit in case of greater than type along the X- axis and corresponding cumulative frequencies along the Y-axis, points are plotted and joined by a free hand (Image 4 and Image 5). Class limits are actual class limits i.e., continuous distribution.

Steps of Construction

Step1: Prepare class interval and place frequency against it

Step 2: Determine true class limits (upper and lower)

True upper-class limit=1/2(upper score limit of the respective interval +lower score limit of next higher interval)

True lower-class limit=1/2(lower score limit of the respective interval +upper score limit of previous interval)

Step 3: Insert a column for cumulative frequency (CF)

Step 4: Along X axis plot true upper-class limit in case of Less than Ogive and true lower-class limit in case of Greater than Ogive along with corresponding CF.

Step 5: True lower-class limit of the lowest class interval is also marked on the X axis.

Step 6: Join the plotted points. (Calculation through Excel is easy).

Applications

An ogive is helpful in determining median, mode, mean, quartiles and percentiles accurately. It is helpful for determination of performance of a specific group and overall comparison of groups.

Table 5: Cumulative Frequency Table

Weight	Frequency	CF (Less Than)	CF (More Than)
20-30	6	6	40
30-40	8	14	34
40-50	12	26	26
50-60	10	36	14
60-70	4	40	4

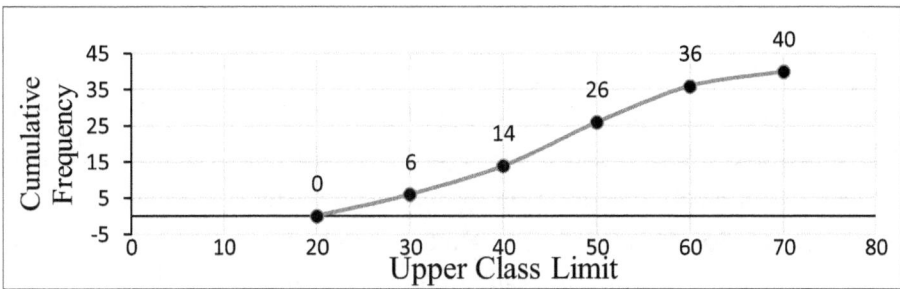

Image 4: Less Than Type Ogive

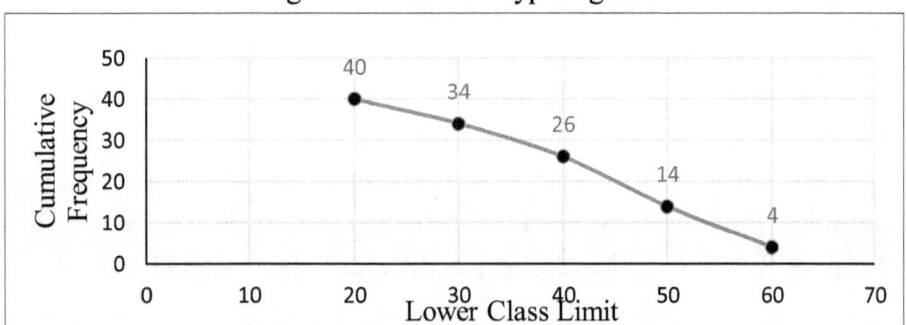

Image 5: Greater Than Type Ogive

Box and Whisker Plot

It is a graphical representation of numerical data. Before going to the details of this plot, we will first focus on some basics of methods of presenting different kinds of data presentation. Data are presented either in graphical or table form. Initially from raw data, frequency distribution table is prepared, and after that we go for graphical presentation. Now there are different methods of presentation and it depends on the nature of data.

There are two types of data: one is qualitative and other is quantitative. Quantitative data is of two types: discrete numerical and continuous. Pie chart is for qualitative, Bar chart for both qualitative and discrete numerical (quantitative). Histogram summarizes continuous numerical whereas Dot plot for discrete numerical. Histogram uses bars similar to bar chart but there remains no gap between bars to indicate its continuous nature. Another wonderful method is Stem and leaf plot combining both table and diagram. Box and whisker plot is another graphical method that helps us to present large set of numerical data easily.

Features of Box-Whisker Plot: Box and whisker plot is based five summary values. Minimum value, Q1 (first quartile/25th percentile/lower quartile), Q2 (median/25th percentile/middle quartile), Q3 (third quartile 75th percentile/upper quartile), maximum value. In addition, outliers are shown with dots/asterisks (Image 6). After calculating all the summary values, a rectangle (vertical or horizontal) is drawn extending from Q1 to Q3, and Q2 or median dividing the rectangle but may not be symmetrical. A line or whisker starts from either side of box and joins minimum and maximum value; usually whisker is not greater than 1.5times the IQR. IQR is defined as difference between Q3 and Q1.

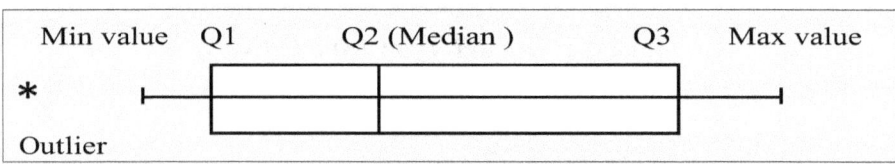

Image 6: Box -Whisker Plot

Construction of Box - Whisker plot
Step 1: Arrange data in ascending order
Step 2: Consider data contains even or odd numbered values
Step 3: Calculate median first
Step 4: Calculate Q1 &Q3
Step 5: Calculate IQ range
Step 6: Identify Minimum & Maximum value
Step 7: Construct a scale that includes entire range of data
Step 8: Draw a rectangle whose arms represent Q1 & Q3
Step 9: Whiskers drawn as described above
Step 10: Outliers with asterisks shown

Applications of Box-Whisker Plot
- Large set of data can easily be presented
- Multiple data set comparison when arranged side by side
- Outliers can be detected
- Nature of distribution can be assessed
- Overall view of dispersion of data

Histogram

Frequency distribution of continuous quantitative variable is presented graphically in two ways: Frequency polygon and Histogram. Histogram consists of consecutive bars without any gap. This indicates the continuous nature of the dataset. Base (along X axis) represents length of class interval and height (along Y axis) corresponds to frequency (Image 7). Cases in a particular class interval are uniformly distributed over the class interval whereas in frequency polygon, cases are located at the midpoint of class interval. Frequency polygon is a line graph where frequencies of class intervals are plotted against midpoint of each class interval. This is helpful for comparison of frequency distribution of more than one set of data where histogram is not suitable. Histogram is a versatile tool for identifying nature of data distribution, detects skewness and presence of an outlier. It gives insight about data spread and measures of central tendency.

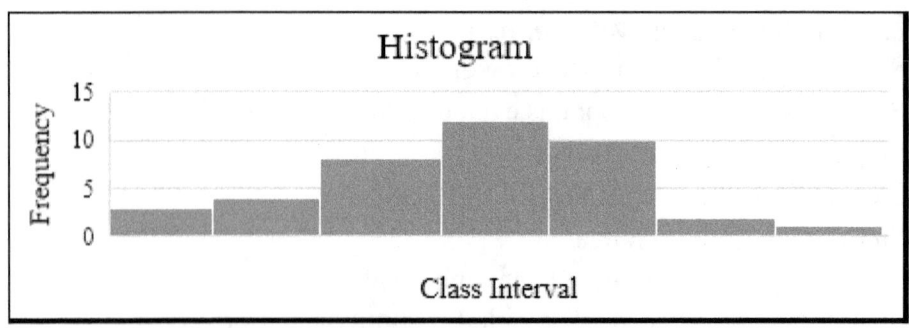

Image 7: Histogram

How to determine number and width of Class Interval in Histogram?
Suppose following is the data set: 2,3,5,8,9,12,4,10,14,6
Through data inspection, we get the following information:
Total number of data points (N)=10, Largest value 14, Smallest 2
Step 1: Find range (Here 14-2=12)
$Range$ = Largest Value − Smallest Value
Step 2: Determine number of intervals. Two methods are available. Sturges' formula: Number of intervals= $1 + \log_2 N$ where N is the number of total data points. Here N=10, using this formula this gives 4.3. We may round to 4 or 5 (Usually rounded to next higher integer). Another option is Number of intervals =Square root of Total data points i.e. $\sqrt{10}$ which equals 3.16. So, we may choose 3 or 4 intervals.
Sturges' formula is applied when there is normal distribution. In case of Skewed data or presence of an outlier or small size of sample, formula gives inappropriate results. In such situations, other alternative approaches are available but I am not going to the details. In recent times, students are more comfortable with Excel. But without basic knowledge of construction of a frequency distribution table and preparing class interval, you cannot run excel.
Step 3: Width of class interval is given by the formula
Width= $\frac{Range}{Number\ of\ Class\ Interval} = \frac{12}{4} = 3$ (deciding 4 class intervals)
Step 4: Prepare class intervals
2-4,5-7,8-10,11-13, 14-16 (Number of class intervals adjusted to 5 to include all data points). This is a discrete type of frequency distribution. To avoid gap between class intervals, we will have to make it a

continuous distribution. For that purpose, calculate adjustment factor which is to be subtracted from lower class limit of one class and added to higher class limit to previous class.

Step 5: Adjustment factor is given by the following formula

$$= \frac{Lower\ limit\ of\ one\ class - Upper\ limit\ of\ previous\ class}{2}$$

Step 6: Prepare a table after adjustment (Table 6)

Step 6: Put Class Intervals after adjustment in X axis and corresponding Frequency in Y axis.

Table 6: Class Interval for Histogram

Class Interval before Adjustment	Class Interval after Adjustment
2-4	1.5-4.5
5-7	4.5-7.5
8-10	7.5-10.5
11-13	10.5-13.5
14-16	13.5-16.5

Tabular Method of Presentation

Statistical Table

Table is a structured format containing rows and columns for presenting quantitative data. Tabular presentation helps us to understand data easily. Analysis and comparison become easy. Huge amount of information can be easily presented in a table. Statistical Table has two main parts - Horizontal rows and Vertical columns. In construction of a table, following parts are identified (Image 3):

- Table number
- Table Title
- Head note below title contain information about title
- Row and Column caption: Heading of each row and Column
- Stub: Main heading of rows
- Box head: Main heading of columns
- Body: Main part consists of cells containing information.
- Foot note is placed just below table (usually identified as in the form of *, +, @ seen in the table not explained) and gives explanations and additional information about data.
- Source note below foot note indicates sources of information

Biostatistics in Health Research

Follow journal policy for presentation of results of research. Ideally there should be no vertical lines, and only three horizontal lines-one below title, one below column head and at the bottom of the table.

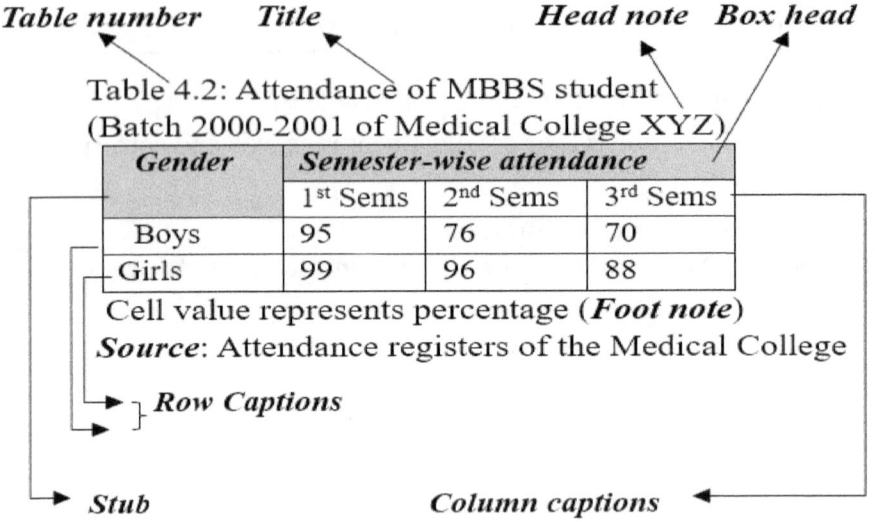

Image 3: Statistical Table

Test your understanding

1. What is a statistical table? Write different parts of a statistical table with a diagram.
2. What is Class limit and Class Interval?
3. What are the different types of Class Interval? Give example for each.
4. What are the different types of Frequency Distribution Table?
5. What is Sturges' formula? Where is it applicable?
6. What are the limitations of Sturges' formula? How to deal with these situations?
7. What is adjustment factor? When is it used?
8. What is Stub and Box Head?
9. Write two uses of Box and Whisker plot.

Section 6: Distribution of Data

Discrete probability distribution
Binomial, Geometric, Hypergeometric, Poisson, Negative binomial,
Continuous probability distribution
Normal, Chi-squared, t-distribution, F-distribution, Exponential

Normal Distribution

It is very common in biomedical research. After data collection, if we draw histogram after plotting frequency in Y axis against data interval in X axis and join the midpoints of bars of histogram, we get bell-shaped curve also known as Normal distribution. We can easily draw a bell-shaped curve with excel function NORM.DIST(x, mean, standard deviation, FALSE). After calculating mean and SD, go to insert tab and then scatter with smooth line after selecting score and probability mass function (Image 8).

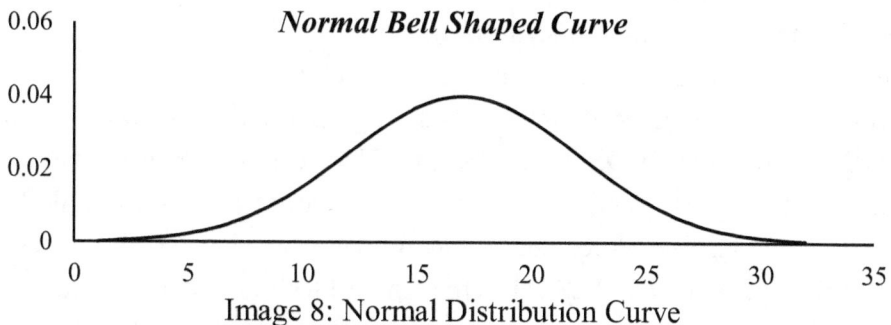

Image 8: Normal Distribution Curve

Features of Normal Curve
- ❖ Unimodal, bell shaped
- ❖ Symmetrical about mean (Mean, median and mode coincide)
- ❖ Area under the curve is 1.
- ❖ Flattens symmetrically as variance increases but tails never touch baseline in horizontal axis

Standard normal distribution is a special type of normal distribution where mean equal zero and SD equals I. Each point in the data set is represented by Z score and standardized so that comparison becomes easy (standardized). Z score have been discussed later on.

Poisson Distribution

This is a type of discrete distribution where sample size is large, but probability of a particular event is very small. Here we express the probability of a given number of rare events occurring in a fixed interval (of space, time, volume or area). It assumes a normal distribution when mean becomes larger. In Poisson distribution, sample size is definite, and we know the probability of events.

Assumptions
- Events are occurring at random
- Events are independent of each other
- They are occurring at a uniform rate

Properties
- Discrete type of distribution
- Expresses probability of *Number* of Rare Events
- Skewed to right, Leptokurtic
- Mean equals variance (most important character)

Mathematics of Poisson Distribution

If the average occurrence of a particular rare event is λ (lambda), then probability of r number of rare events during a particular interval is given by the formula: $P(r, \lambda) = (\lambda^r * e^{-\lambda})/r!$. Here e is the base of natural logarithm (e=2.718) and r! –pronounce as factorial r (as an example 5! = 5*4*3*2*1). We can calculate this probability using Excel function POISSON.DIST(r, λ, FALSE/TRUE) where TRUE instructs cumulative and FALSE instructs to put particular probability of that number of events only. We may also take help of free online Graph pad software. Another common inference to report in a study result is calculation of CI. $CI = L \pm (t \times \sqrt{L})$ where L is the average count. Remember *Mean = Variance*, and $SEM = \frac{SD}{\sqrt{n}}$. t value depends on level of significance.

Application

Rare events may be mental retardation, chromosomal abnormalities, suicide rate. In real life situation, we first estimate probability of a rare events using Poisson probability. And after implementation of a preventive measure (say health program) again we estimate its probability using same principle. Finally, we apply Chi-square test to see the difference. Thus, Poisson theory is applicable in two situations: estimation of number of rare events probability or burden of rare events and other is effectiveness of a program.

Problem1: Compute the probability of occurrence of three cases of Down syndrome in a sample of 750 children from a population having 0.4% incidence of that disorder.

Go to Excel-Formula -Statistical functions then find
POISSON.DIST(x, mean, cumulative) where
X: The number of events.
Mean: The expected numeric value.
Cumulative: TRUE, returns the cumulative Poisson probability of the events occurring will be between zero and x inclusive; if FALSE, it returns the Poisson probability will be exactly x.
Here Mean = (0.4/100) *750=3, X=3
Cumulative: True (This means probability of cases may be 0,1,2,3 then to be added). Putting all these arguments in POISSON.DIST(x, mean, cumulative), we get 64.7% probability.

Binomial Distribution

In binomial distribution, sample size is definite, and we know the probability of events. There are two possible outcomes or events. In each trial or experiment, two outcomes are mutually exclusive. Probability of each event is fixed in each trial and probability of each event is constant from trial to trial. Events or outcomes are not affected by the outcome of any other trial. Here sample size is large, but probability of a particular event is very small. Here we express the probability of a given number of rare events occurring in a fixed interval (of space, time, volume or area). It assumes a normal distribution when mean becomes larger.

Assumptions
- Events are occurring at random
- Events are independent of each other
- Probability of each event is fixed in each trial
- Probability of each event is constant from trial to trial

Properties
- Discrete type of distribution
- Mean = np, Variance = npq
- When p = 0.05, distribution is symmetric

Mathematics of Binomial Distribution

We can calculate this probability using Excel function BINOMDIST (number_s, trial, probability_s, TRUE/FALSE) where TRUE instructs cumulative and FALSE instructs to put particular probability of that number of events only. We may also take help of free online Graph pad software. (www.graphpad.com/quickcalc/).

Application of binomial and Poisson theory depends on the frequency of outcome. If outcome is rare and population is huge, go for Poisson. But when the sample size is finite and outcome is not rare, go for Binomial distribution. Remember in both types of distributions, outcome is dichotomized, and we find the probability of number of particular outcomes. Chi-square distribution usually deals with 2* 2 contingency table, two variables where each variable is binary. As Chi- square distribution is continuous, some corrections are necessary for such situation of contingency table known as Yate's correction.

Problem1: Suppose a disease has got 2% mortality, if I take 30 people for my study, is the sample size is adequate?

Take Home Messages
- We don't have to calculate manually
- We don't have to remember formula
- We have Excel function BINOM.DIST/ POISSON.DIST(r, λ, FALSE/TRUE)
- We have online Graph pad software which is free (www.graphpad.com/quickcalc/)

Section 7: Data Transformation

The pattern of values of a variable is known as a distribution of data. It may be normal or non-normal. It is essential to detect skewed/normal distributions.

Objectives of Data Transformation
- Make the data to follow normal distribution
- Makes analysis and interpretation easy
- Facilitates comparison

Simple Ways to Detect Skewness (Image 9)
- Mean < 2SD-Skewness present
- Graphical method-Histogram
- Normality testing by Kolmogorov - Smirnov test

Common Rules of Data Transformation
- SD is proportional to mean- Logarithmic
- Variance proportional to the mean-Square Root Transformation. Common in cases of count data.
- SD proportional to the mean squared- Reciprocal transformation (serum creatinine -highly variable)

Reporting Section
- Statistical analyses of the transformed data
- Summary of the raw data and Reason for transformation
- Back transformation value with 95% CI

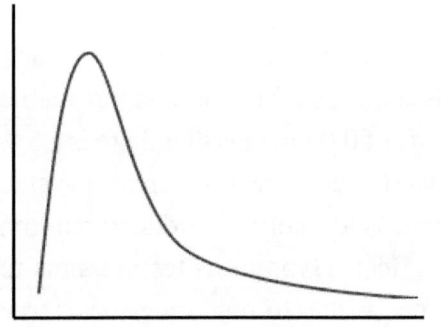   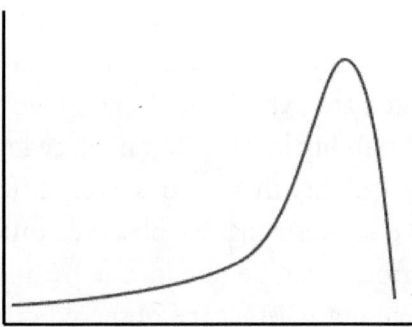

Positively Skewed   Negatively Skewed
Image 9: Asymmetric Distribution

Note: Type of skewness is determined by location of **tail** not its peak

Chapter 3: Hypothesis Testing

Section 1: Hypothesis Testing

Overview

Hypothesis is a statement about population not for sample. During a research process, with the help of sample values we interpret about population parameter. This is known as hypothesis testing. To know the significance of our results of sample, we first have to set up a hypothesis which is about population parameter. It simply means inference about the parameter and is drawn through hypothesis testing from sample values/statistics. At the first step, we state two hypotheses: one is null hypothesis or H_0 and other is known as alternate hypothesis or H_1. Null hypothesis is a hypothesis of no difference. Equality signs ($=, \geq, \leq$) are always attached with it for comparison purpose. In hypothesis testing, null hypothesis is tested as we can calculate the probability of random error/ chance, there is no mathematics for the probability in alternate hypothesis. We test the null hypothesis assuming it is true and test the results of sample by calculating its probability of occurrence by chance or random error. It is judged against α level set before the study. If probability of random error is less than the α level, then we reject null hypothesis and accept alternate hypothesis. Acceptance or rejection of alternate hypothesis depends upon rejection and acceptance of null hypothesis. P value is obtained from the results and is compared with α set before study. Rejection of null hypothesis does not prove but supports alternate hypothesis. Random error is unpredictable and uncontrollable variability in data. Significance level (α) of 0.05 means that there is a 5% probability that the observed difference is due to random error. p-value < α suggests that the observed difference is unlikely to be due to random error, it can be due to true treatment effect. Hypothesis testing aims to find out whether the observed difference is due to random error or true treatment effect. Thus, hypothesis statement will be as follows:

H_0: Treatment is ineffective (difference is due to random error).
H_1: Treatment is effective (unrelated with random error).

Biostatistics in Health Research

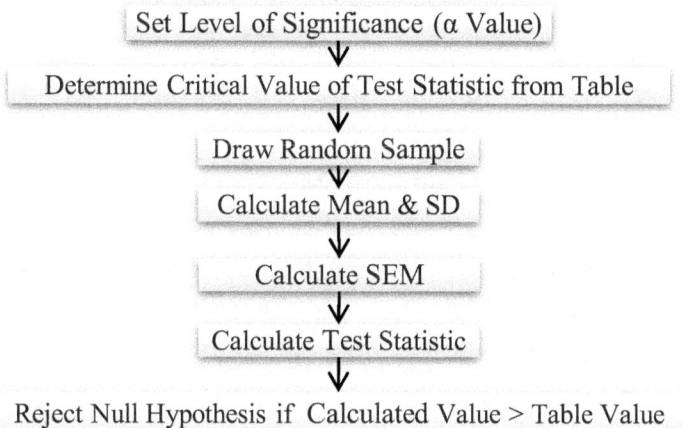

Find Table Value/Critical Value given P-Value and df
t Test one tailed: *T.INV (probability, deg_freedom)*
t Test two tailed: *T.INV.2T (probability, deg_freedom)*

F Test one tailed: *F.INV.RT(probability, deg_freedom1, deg_freedom2)*
F Test two tailed: Adjust p-value and then use *F.INV (probability, deg_freedom1, deg_freedom2)* or *F.INV.RT(probability, deg_freedom1, deg_freedom2)*. Here deg_freedom1 means df for numerator, deg_freedom2 means df for denominator

Chi-square Test one tailed: *CHISQ.INV.RT(probability, deg_freedom)*
Chi-square Test two tailed: Adjust p-value and then use *CHISQ.INV (probability, deg_freedom) or CHISQ.INV.RT(probability, deg_freedom)*

Problem 1: Find table value of Chi-square in 2*2 contingency table given ($P = 0.05$, one tailed test, df=1)=CHISQ.INV.RT(0.05,1) =3.84

Critical Value or Table Value: Sample data gives value of test statistic. Critical value depends on type of test that determines the distribution of test statistics under H_0, tail of test and α. Distribution of test statistic is known from statistical principle and is fixed across samples, this helps to calculate the likelihood of observing the test statistic when H_0 is true. Distribution of sample data varies across samples, so not used in calculating critical value.

Section 2: Terms Related to Hypothesis Testing

Type I and Type II Error

In hypothesis testing, we calculate test statistics and find out its probability from statistical table. With this probability, we can explore whether true effect exists in population or not to a certain degree of confidence. In true sense, there may or may not be an effect in reality. Associated probability of test statistic tells us which is more likely. Even when we are 95% confident with the effect, there is 5% chance where we get effect when no treatment effect exists. Type I error or alpha error or false positive conclusion result when we reject null hypothesis though it is true i.e., we get treatment effect when there is no difference. Type II error or beta error or false negative conclusion occurs when we fail to reject null hypothesis though it is false. In type II error, we conclude no effect though in reality there is difference (Table 1). There is trade-off between these two errors, when one increases other decreases. Nature of relationship is left to researcher to make an educated guess.

Table 1: Errors in Hypothesis Testing

Decision	State of Reality	
	H_0 True	H_0 False
Reject H_0	Type I error	Correct decision
Retain H_0	Correct decision	Type II error

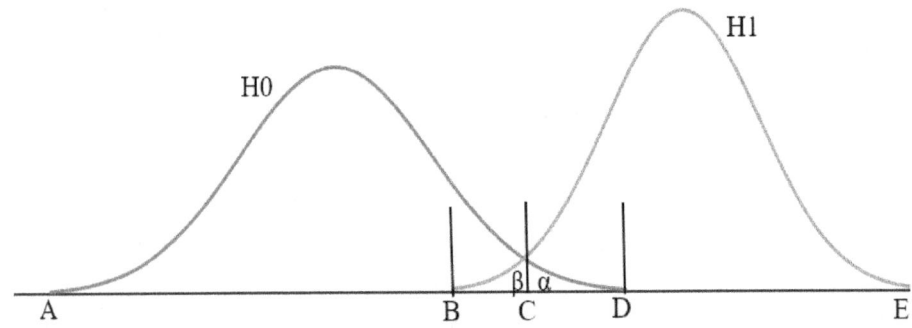

Image 1: Type I and Type II Error

Take it easy through diagram
Left curve corresponds to H_0 and includes area (AD) and Right curve corresponds to H_1 and includes area (BE). With this confidence limit as shown in image 1, we will reject any values right to line C, though these values actually belong to H_0. This is Type I error or α error. Similarly, with this confidence limit, we will accept any values left to line C, though these values actually belong to H_1. This is Type II error or β error. Again, with this confidence limit, values between CE are correctly rejected. This is power of the test. If total area under H_1 is 1, then (1-β) will be power of the study. Power of the study is to correctly reject H_0 in favor of H_1, when H_0 is false. From image 1, it is obvious that both errors cannot be reduced at the same time.

One Tailed and Two Tailed Tests

One Tailed Test
When a researcher begins an experiment with specific prediction about direction of treatment effect. Here H_0 and H_1 specify direction of treatment effect. Critical region/area of rejection is located in one end or tail of the distribution. So, we evaluate specific outcome in one direction and this directional statement is incorporated in both.
Hypothesis statement
H_0: Mean BP is not reduced and H_1: Mean BP is reduced

Two Tailed Test
When a researcher begins an experiment without specific prediction about direction of treatment effect. Here H_0 and H_1 specify no direction of treatment effect. Critical region or area of rejection is located in both ends and tails of the distribution. So, we cannot introduce specific direction of outcome into the statement of H_0 and H_1. In most of the study, we are not certain in advance, the direction of effect and we allow for either eventuality.
Hypothesis statement
H_0: Mean BP is not altered with anti-hypertensive agent
H_1: Mean BP is altered with anti-hypertensive agent

Power of a Study

Ability of a test to reject a false null hypothesis. In type II error, false null hypothesis is accepted. It is expressed in terms of probability i.e., ability to detect a true treatment effect. Conventionally the power of study is kept at 0.8 which means 80% chance of detecting the difference when there is true treatment effect. $Power = 1 - Type\ II\ error\ (\beta)$.

Factors affecting Power of a Study (See Image 2)

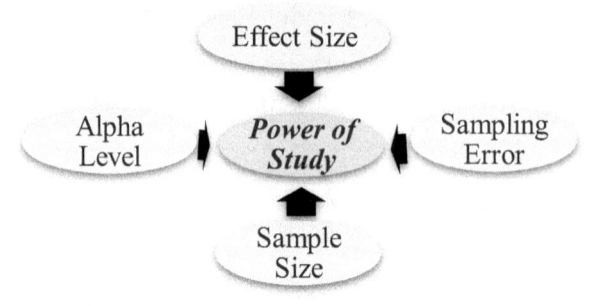

Image 2: Factors Affecting Power of a Study

When sample size is increased, sampling error decreased ($SE = SD/\sqrt{sample\ size}$). If error is decreased, effect size is increased. Effect size is also increase when there is large difference between means. We know, $Effect\ size = Difference\ in\ Means\ /SE$. Most practical way to increase the power of a test is to increase the sample size. Remember when alpha level increases, rejection of null hypothesis is more likely but there should be trade-off between type I and type II error as type II error decreases only when type I error increases. We know, $Power = 1 - Type\ II\ error$. So, power of the study increased. Thus, calculation of power is a complex procedure which investigator should keep in mind.

Confidence Interval (CI)

It is a good estimate of population parameter. This is an interval which is constructed from each sample values when we take samples from population. We can construct confidence interval for each sample. Confidence level states the percentage of confidence intervals that contain true population value (It is to mention here that confidence interval indicates the likelihood that a result will fall within the stated limit whereas significance level tells us the probability/likelihood of result falling outside the stated limit or range). Usually 95%, 99% confidence levels are used. 95% confidence level means – if we take 100 samples, construct confidence interval for each, then 95% of intervals will contain population parameter. Remember do not attach the term probability to population parameter as it is a constant value. Confidence limits are the two boundaries of the interval.

Concepts behind CI

If we take repeated samples from population, in each sample, we will get mean and SD. It can be shown that means of the samples will follow normal distribution. Mean of all these means of samples closely approximates population mean but sample SD is not representative of population SD. In reality, we do not collect many samples, but one large sample (observations more than 30) is taken and is supposed to be representative of population. We made a correction on SD of that sample and that is known as Standard error of mean (SEM) and is expressed as $SEM = SD/\sqrt{Sample\ Size}$. Now we are in a possession to construct an interval estimate (CI) of population parameter with the help of SEM.

Steps of Construction

Step 1- One large sample (observations more than 30) is taken
Step 2- Calculate mean
Step 3- Calculate SD
Step 4- Calculate SEM ($SEM = SD/\sqrt{sample\ size}$)
Step 5- Find Z value when sample is large or t value when small.
Then construct interval for single mean or proportions:
CI=Mean±(Z×SEM) (For large sample) .... (1)
CI=Mean±(t×SEM) (For small sample) .... (2)
CI for proportion=$p \pm \left(Z \times \frac{\sqrt{pq}}{n}\right)$ .... (3)
When two samples mean or proportions:
CI for diff in mean=Diff±[Z×SE(Diff)] .... (4)
CI for diff in proportion=$(p_1-p_2) \pm \left[1.96 \times \sqrt{\frac{p_1q_1}{n_1} + \frac{p_2q_2}{n_2}}\right]$ .... (5)
(Where p is proportion of characteristic, $q = 1 - p$). Thus, with the help

of sample values, we can construct an interval known as CI that includes population parameter. In similar way, we estimate CI of most population parameters (OR and r).

Factors affecting CI *(Image 3)*

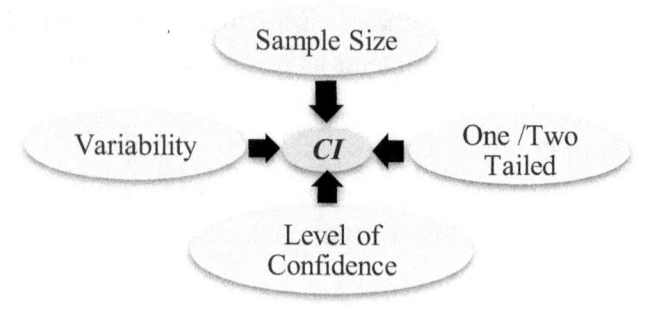

Image 3: Factors Affecting CI

Application of CI
- Estimating interval for population parameter in which it lies
- Hypothesis testing- commonly our decision in hypothesis testing depends on p-value and level of significance. In similar way, we may reject null hypothesis or accept alternate hypothesis based on the calculated CI using same significance level whether a particular value specified in null hypothesis falls within this range or outside this range.

Test Your Concept
1. Level of confidence is 90%, Can you say that there is 90% probability that a population parameter will be included in CI?
2. When two CIs of two independent samples overlap and do not overlap, what will be your conclusion?

Explore Your Statistical Knowledge
- ✓ Misinterpretation of CI
- ✓ Misinterpretation of P-value
- ✓ Misinterpretation of results of Hypothesis Testing

Effect Size

In a hypothesis testing, if we get test statistic which is significant does not necessarily mean that effect is important. We are least interested about statistical significance. We should measure the effect in a standardized way. Larger the effect size more is the observed effect.

Measuring the effect in a standardized manner is known as effect size. It is the quantitative measure of treatment effect. Standardization helps to compare different variables across various studies and also when different scales of measurements are used. It is thus useful and provides us importance of effect size.

Table 2: Effect Size in Different Types of Analysis

Type of Test	Effect Size
Student t test	Cohen's d
Chi-square test	Odds Ratio
Correlation	Correlation Coefficient
ANOVA/Regression	Partial eta squared

Examples ((Table 2)
- ❖ Cohen's d- measures effect size for the comparison between two means. It can be used in t-test and ANOVA results and also in meta-analysis. Cohen considered $d = 0.2$ as small effect size, $d = 0.5$ as medium effect size and 0.8 as large effect size.

$$\text{Cohen's d} = \frac{\text{Difference in Means Between Groups}}{\text{Standard Deviation}}$$

- ❖ Correlation coefficient (r)- gives us measure of strength of relationship between two variables. Its value ranges between 0 and 1.
- ❖ OR- used when data are binary in nature and compares odds of an effect (success) in treatment group to that in control.
- ❖ Eta square which is also an effect size reflects the variance in dependent variable explained by independent variable.

Test Statistics

Test statistics tells us how good our hypothesis explains the data against what it cannot explain. There are two types of variation: one is systematic error or variation and other is unsystematic or random error or chance. To test whether our hypothesis is a good explanation of the data, we compare systematic error with that of unsystematic or random error or chance. Systematic error represents variance explained by the model whereas unsystematic error represents variance not explained by the model. After calculating the statistic value, we can calculate its probability from statistical table. This allows us to establish how likely it would be that we would get a test statistic of a certain size if there were no effect (i.e., the null hypothesis was true).

The exact form of this equation changes depending on which test statistic calculating, but the important thing to be that they all represent the same thing: the amount of variance explained compared to the variance that can't be explained by the model. We know many statistics such as t, F, χ^2 used in t test, ANOVA and Chi-square test. P value obtained from the results is compared with α set before study. If it is less than α, we reject null hypothesis and conclude that real treatment effect exists. Value of test statistics differ whether it is one-tailed or two tailed. We can calculate it manually or using excel function (Go to excel-Formula-Statistical function and then choose the function)

$$\text{Test statistic} = \frac{\text{Variance explained by the model}}{\text{Variance not explained by the model}} = \frac{\text{Treatment effect}}{\text{Random error}}$$

Commonly Used Test Statistics in Biomedical Research

- ❖ $\text{t statistic} = \dfrac{\text{Mean difference}}{\text{Standard error of mean}}$

- ❖ $\text{F statistic} = \dfrac{\text{Between groups variation}}{\text{Within groups variation}}$

- ❖ $\chi^2 = \sum \dfrac{(\text{Observed frequency} - \text{Expected frequency})^2}{\text{Expected frequency}}$

P-Value

It is defined as the probability of occurrence of an observed effect due to chance or random error. This probability reflects the measure of evidence against the null hypothesis. It indicates how likely the result of our research is when null hypothesis is true.

P-value is obtained from sample. Whether a result is significant or not is based on whether p-value is less or more than the level of significance (α level) which is decided by the investigator before data collection. Value of α is arbitrary and depends on decision of researcher. P-value and α value both are expressed in terms of probability. When P-value is greater than alpha, result is not significant and when smaller than α, result is significant. P-value is the maximum probability of obtaining the outcome by random error/chance. P value is **not related with probability** of null hypothesis; it is related with the null hypothesis. To simplify once again, during analysis of data from sample, our idea is to find the probability of results due to random error. Alpha value decided before the study proper tells us criteria to reject or accept null hypothesis. The probability of effect observed in the study, if less than or equal to α, null hypothesis will be rejected. Usually, it is fixed at a level of 0.05. When p value is less than or equal to 0.05, result is significant (null hypothesis is rejected). Suppose that a sleeping pill study produced a P value of 0.03. This P value indicates that if the pill had no effect, we obtain the difference or more in 3% of cases due to random error. If we reject the hypothesis, then we are wrong in 3% of cases as we have decided beforehand that probability of α < 0.05 means significant. We are considering probability of random error below 0.05 is significant.

Problem with P-Value

It is now clear that at the end of study, researcher classifies the result as significant or not. He decides on the basis of p-value whether it is less than or equal to α, if so, null hypothesis is rejected and result is statistically significant. When obtained p- value is > α, result is not significant. When α is set to 0.05, we are still wrong in 5% of cases assuming null hypothesis is true. 0.05 level of significance is merely a convention, it does not imply that result on other side is necessarily different This is one problem with p-value.

Non-significant p value is due to small sample size and we may be wrong in our decision when null hypothesis is rejected. Again, statistically significant result may or may not be clinically significant. So, consider clinical effect of observed result before accepting alternate hypothesis or rejecting null hypothesis. Frequently misinterpretation of p value is another problem. P value mainly tells us the result whether significant or not. Range of values in outcome is not considered which is required for meaningful interpretation. To overcome the limitations of p value, CI is being used to report results of a study. As it is expressed in interval, confidence is much more than p value. Considering all these aspects, p value along with CI is better than p value alone. In recent times, scientific community is worried about the reproducibility and replicability of results based on p values. Some journal has banned the use of p-value.

Find P Value using Excel Function

T.TEST (array1, array2, tails, type)
Array1-The first data set., Array 2-The second data set
Tails: 1=one tailed and 2=two tailed
Type S1 for paired sampled, 2 for Independent sample (Equal variances) and 3 for Independent sample (Unequal variances)

CHISQ.TEST(actual_range,expected_range)
actual -Observed frequencies, expected -Expected frequencies range

Z.TEST (array,x,[sigma]) gives one tailed p value
Array-　range of data against which to test x.
x- The value to test.
σ- population standard deviation (optional). If not known, sample SD is used.

F.TEST (array1, array2) gives two tailed probability
Array1-The first data set., Array2-The second data set.

Section 3: Frequently Asked Questions

1. What is Hypothesis, Thesis and Dissertation?
2. Write different types of research questions with example.
3. What is Probability, Possibility, Likelihood, Chance?
4. Which is the first step in hypothesis testing?
5. Why equality sign is used in statement of Null hypothesis?
6. Why you test Null hypothesis?
7. Give one example of one tailed and two tailed test.
8. Why there is error in hypothesis testing?
9. Does p value have importance if your research involves non-probability method of sampling?
10. Statistical significance versus clinical significance-Discuss.
11. Random error: Significance in research.
12. What is the difference between α value and p- value?
13. What does it mean when P=0.02?
14. What do you mean by CI, Confidence Limit and Confidence Level? Give example for differences with those term.
15. What is Central Limit Theorem?
16. Simply double the p value of one tailed test to get p value of two tailed test: True or False. Justify your decision. Table value
    If the study specifically designed to measure the probability in one direction, then and then you can double to get two tailed p value otherwise it is not correct.
17. What is Critical value/ Table value?
18. Write difference between Critical value and Test Statistic?
19. Are the critical value and test statistic change with the one or two tailed tests?
    Critical value depends on α, type of test (one or two tailed). So, value changes whereas value of test statistic is calculated based on sample data and it remains same.
20. Which excel function is used to calculate CI?
    CONFIDENCE.T(alpha, standard_dev,size)
    CONFIDENCE.NORM(alpha,standard_dev,size)

Chapter 4: Types of Study

Section 1: Different Types of Study

Broadly type of research is classified into three types: Qualitative, Quantitative and Mixed type. Presenting here a flow chart for different types of Quantitative studies (Flow Chart 1-3) and then I shall discuss salient features of them.

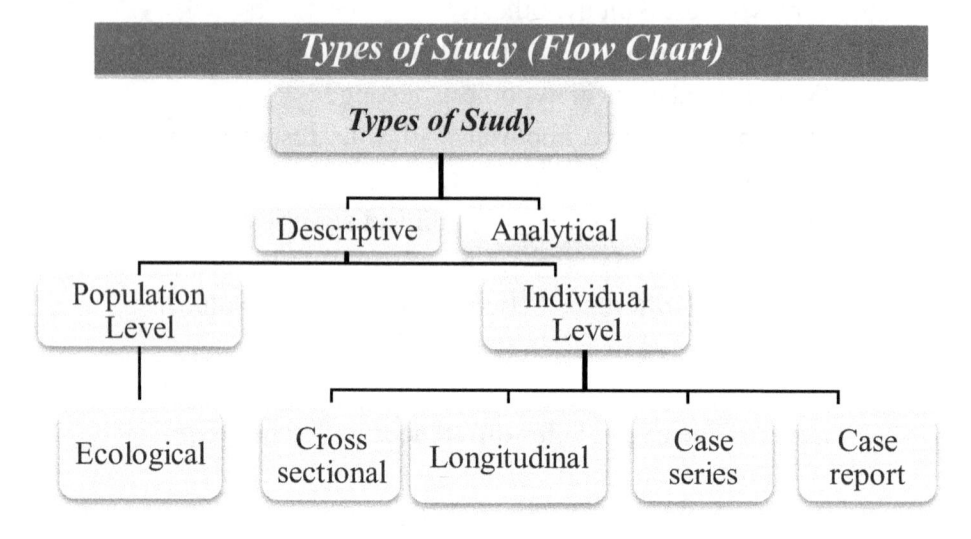

Types of Study (Flow Chart)

```
                    Types of Study
                          |
              ┌───────────┴───────────┐
          Descriptive              Analytical
              |
      ┌───────┴────────────────────────┐
  Population                       Individual
    Level                            Level
      |                                |
  Ecological        ┌──────────┬───────┴──────┬──────────┐
                 Cross     Longitudinal    Case         Case
                sectional                  series       report
```

Flow Chart I: Types of Study (Descriptive)

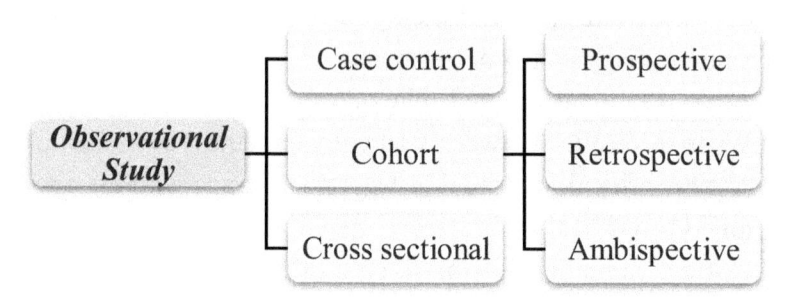

```
                    ┌── Case control ──┬── Prospective
   Observational    |                  |
      Study    ────┼── Cohort ─────────┼── Retrospective
                    |                  |
                    └── Cross sectional└── Ambispective
```

Flow Chart 2: Analytical Study (Observational)

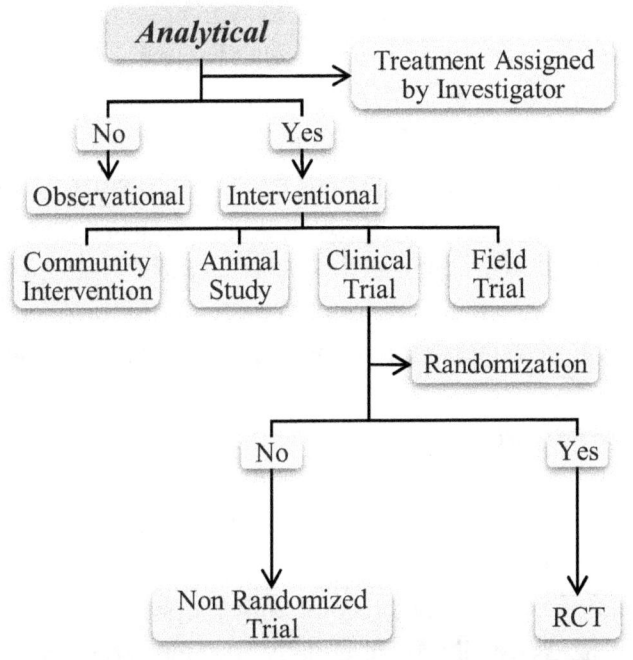

Biostatistics in Health Research

```
                    Analytical ─────► Treatment Assigned
                   ┌────┴────┐              by Investigator
                  No         Yes
                   ▼           ▼
             Observational  Interventional
                    ┌──────┬──────┬──────┐
              Community  Animal  Clinical  Field
              Intervention Study  Trial   Trial
                                    │
                                    ▼
                              Randomization
                             ┌──────┴──────┐
                            No             Yes
                             ▼              ▼
                      Non Randomized       RCT
                          Trial
```

Flow Chart 3: Analytical Study (Interventional)

Qualitative Research

In qualitative research, we try to investigate social reality from participant point of view, their perceptions, meanings and interpretations. It is subjective rather than measuring it objectively from the investigators experience. More often it is concerned to answer the question why and interpretation of responses of the participant. Information is collected in the form of text.

When is it done?
- View social phenomenon
- Subject matter is unfamiliar or insufficiently researched
- Exploring the behaviour and Seeking depth of understanding

Methods of Data Collection

In-Depth (Individual) Interviews: done in case of highly sensitive subject matter. It is an open-ended interview carried out in geographically dispersed areas, not based on pre- structured interview format, level of interview varies according to responses of the participant. We get in-depth information, but results are not generalizable.

Focus Group Discussions (FGD): It is also an open-ended interview and done where group interaction is important. There are six to eight persons with similar various characteristics (homogeneous) are chosen. There should be a predetermined FGD guide. Each session usually not last more than one and half hour and 2-3 sessions are considered sufficient for each population subgroup. Moderator and Note taker are there, audio visual recording done. This method can identify problems and goals, and helps to evaluate an intervention. We get lot of information in a short period of time in comparison to in-depth interview. Results are not generalizable.

Participant Observations: Researcher himself becomes participant in the study; it is hard to take notes and recordings. Data are deep and detailed. Analysis of the data is challenging and still evolving.

Sampling Methods

Non-probability sampling method commonly purposive sampling method is used. Sample size is usually small. Usually, sampling continues until no new information is generated. Number of subjects in the sample is not known before the research starts.

Analysis

Grounded theory: Understanding data and developing theories.

Content analysis: Starts with the theoretical framework and then analyses the data to understand the theory.

Qualitative research may be forerunner of quantitative research. Sometimes both methods of research are carried out simultaneously or qualitative method is done after quantitative research. We try to triangulate to check the hypothesis.

Disadvantages

It is time consuming; documentation depends on memory of researcher and requires much effort to achieve its objective. Qualitative research method describes individual experience and inductive not deductive in nature, it does not measure the level of confidence and cannot predict causal relationship.

Software in Qualitative Research

Software packages for qualitative analysis available which can code the information quickly and efficiently but cannot determine meaningful categories through coding and analyze the factors of interest. Software packages should be discouraged for such type of research for exploring in-depth understanding of behavior.

Ecological Study

Ecological Study is a type of descriptive study where group of subjects is unit of study and establishes whether high rate of suspected exposure is related with higher frequency of outcome. It generates hypothesis. Drawback is that individual level information not available. So, interpret with caution to avoid misleading conclusion. Examples include finding relationship of oil consumption of a country with prevalence of heart disease. Still, we perform this type of study when huge amount of information over a large geographical region is almost impossible to collect at individual level. After doing this type of study, we may have confidence and our hypothesis becomes stronger and directs us to conduct a well -designed study such as cohort or case control study for testing hypothesis. It can also be of two types, cross-sectional or longitudinal. If we look at the table 1 below, value of (a + b), (a + c) are known but other parameters are not known, this is why it is also known as incomplete design.

Table 1: Ecological Study Result

	Disease	No Disease	Total
Exposed	a	b	a + b
Unexposed	c	d	c + d
Total	a + c	b + d	a +b +c +d

Case Control Study

Case control study is an observational analytical study where there are comparison groups. Here researcher starts study by picking up cases (presence of outcome of interest) and controls (similar in all respects with the cases except the factor of interest). Usually, incident cases not the prevalent cases are recruited to avoid survival bias for the purpose of the study. Diseases with rapid onset and outcome as in infectious diseases are chosen. Controls are best selected from the population which gave rise to cases. After selection of cases and controls, exposure history elicited. Finally, comparing outcome in exposed groups in both cases and control gives us clue for association. Refer to Table 1 and Flow Chart 4, we get following information:

Steps of Calculation of OR

Step 1: Odds of Exposure among Cases

$$= \frac{\text{Probability of Exposure among Cases}}{\text{Probability of Non- exposure among Cases}}$$

$$= \frac{a}{a+c} \div \frac{c}{a+c} = \frac{a}{c}$$

Step 2: Odds of Exposure among Controls $= \frac{b}{d}$

Step 3: Odds Ratio in Case Control Study

$$= \frac{\text{Odds of Exposure among Cases}}{\text{Odds of Exposure among Controls}} = \frac{a}{c} \div \frac{b}{d} = \frac{ad}{bc}$$

Nature of variables i.e., scale of measurement may differ in exposure or outcome variable which determines the statistical test to be carried out in analysis stage. Subjects are selected either by systematic random sampling technique as the cases occur or by simple random sampling method when all cases have occurred. Biases may occur which may be selection bias or information bias. Potential confounding factors if any are adjusted at design stage.

Case control study takes less time to carry out, suitable for rare diseases, less expensive and there is no attrition problem. This type of study is not suitable where exposure is rare.

Analysis depends upon nature of data. Chi-square test considering binary nature of the data are carried out. OR and CI are reported. If the outcome is continuous nature, t test is performed. Association of lung cancer and smoking are best described with this type of study design. Two important situations where case control study is conducted: Rare outcome and when randomization not possible.

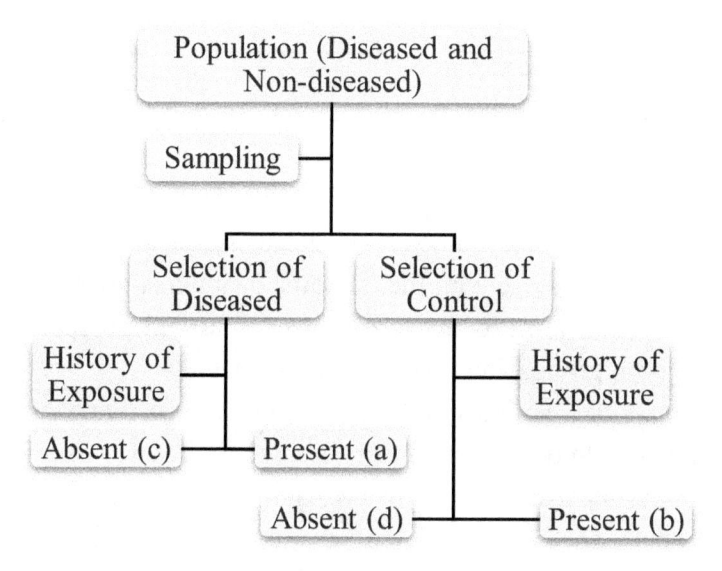

```
          Population (Diseased and
              Non-diseased)
                   │
               Sampling
        ┌──────────┴──────────┐
   Selection of          Selection of
    Diseased               Control
        │                     │
   History of            History of
    Exposure              Exposure
        │                     │
   Absent (c) ── Present (a)
              Absent (d) ── Present (b)
```

Flow Chart 4: Case Control Study

Cohort Study

Cohort study is an observational analytical study where investigator does not assign any exposure and is preferred as it is very strong design (presence of comparison group and prospective in nature).

Strength of the Study
- Very good and strong design compared to other observational study
- Ideal for studying rare exposure
- Temporal relationship can be established (Relative Risk)
- Many outcomes for a give exposure can be evaluated

Weakness
- Time consuming and requires large sample size
- Expensive not suitable for rare outcome
- Attrition problem

Bias

Any type of biases may occur but biases due attrition problem, ascertainment bias and bias from observer point of view is very likely. As during recruitment, all subjects are assessed by researcher for exposure status, recall bias is less.

Calculation of Relative Risk (Table 1)

$$\text{Relative risk} = \frac{\text{Incidence of disease among exposed}}{\text{Incidence of disease among nonexposed}} = \frac{[a/(a+b)]}{[c/(c+d)]}$$

$RR = 1$ means No Association, >1 means Positively Associated and <1 means Negatively Associated.

Types of Cohort Study

Prospective Cohort - at the time of study, subjects are assessed for exposure status and those with the outcome of interest are excluded.

Then exposed and nonexposed groups are observed prospectively for outcome in both groups and relative risk estimated.

A physiologist decided to conduct a study to investigate association between exercise and coronary heart disease. He defined exercise as 45 min continuous walking/jogging or cycling in a day for 5 days in a week. Coronary heart disease is outcome here and specified as ST segment changes. Subjects included 30-50years. He selected 200 subjects in one group and they are not doing exercise and another group of 200 subjects are taking exercises.

Both groups were screened for CAD before start of the study and subjects having ST segment changes were excluded from the study. Now both groups are followed up over a period of 10 years. Then each individual in both groups were screened for ECG changes. Association between ECG changes and exercise is determined.

Retrospective Cohort - At the start of study, outcome is present.

Based on the suspected or possible risk factor, we divide the population into two groups –exposed and non- exposed available on health record. So, in this type of study, exposure and outcome have already occurred. Now we search for outcome on exposed and non- exposed group and calculate incidence of outcome- in both exposed and unexposed group. Odds ratio provides an estimate of relative risk in this type of study. Requires less time, less expensive and suited for rare outcome but the study has no control over exposure, outcome and confounding factor.

Using cancer registry of a hospital, a researcher collected data on chemical exposure of workers and bladder carcinoma on patients admitted between 1990 and 2005. Patients were classified as exposed who had history of working in dye industry and others as unexposed. He then compared the frequency of bladder carcinoma among the exposed and the unexposed.

Ambispective Cohort- Preexisting data, documents and health records are obtained for future monitoring. At the start of study, initial information about risk factors is gathered from records and then the groups with and without exposure are followed prospectively. Especially suited for exposures which have both short- and long-term effects also in emergency situation like epidemics where data are collected retrospectively for the study.

An ambispective cohort study regarding idiopathic intracranial hypertension in young patients to predict poor visual outcome was done after 6 months of presentation. Rest of the patients followed up to 6 months. Vision diminution was tested as poor predictor.

Cross Sectional Study

Cross sectional study is an observational study where cross section of the population is studied at one point in time. It may be descriptive or analytical type. In descriptive type, there is no comparison group and no hypothesis testing. In analytical study, there is a control group. After taking a sample, we find out the cases who have the outcome of interest and from the same sample, we then find out who are not diseased. Here the subjects are examined once. If we look at the case control study, investigator take cases from the population and then selects subjects as control from the same source of population from which cases sampled. One thing to note here that there is also a term longitudinal cross - sectional study which includes prospective cohort and interventional study. Here, control represents same population that gave cases also.

Variables
Outcome and exposure variable may be qualitative or quantitative (discrete or continuous).

Sampling
In hospital-based study, take systematic random sample or nonprobability sample preferably consecutive sample. Better go for multistage sampling if community-based study.

Data Analysis
Both variables qualitative and binary in nature, Chi-square test with or

one of the variables is quantitative, do t test and when both are numerical, it is the objective to find out correlation between the two.

Bias

We may face all 3 types of biases. Common biases are survival bias, recall bias and confounding bias.

Applications
- ❖ Measure prevalence and with the idea of prevalence, we can say whether the problem is rare or not
- ❖ Understand distribution - time, place, person
- ❖ Understand the effectiveness of interventions
- ❖ To generate hypothesis and hypothesis testing and may be the starting point of cohort study
- ❖ Find correlation between two continuous variables

Advantages
- ➤ Study takes less time
- ➤ Procedure is easy
- ➤ Cost is less with respect to other design
- ➤ We can plan health care service delivery
- ➤ Helps in disease control

Disadvantages
- ❖ Large sample size, not suitable for study of rare disease
- ❖ Tremendous work load
- ❖ Huge logistic support
- ❖ Cannot establish causality

Clinical Trial (Phase 0)

Clinical trial is the gold standard method for drug development process. Generally, it goes through an extensive procedure from Phase I to Phase IV with numerous numbers of patient involvement, regulatory monitoring and financial burden. But the outcome is not always successful and attrition rate is also high. In 2006, USFDA has introduced this Phase 0 stage of clinical trial which is also called as Micro dosing study phase. The name is such as it occurs between preclinical phase and Phase 1 of study. The official name is given as exploratory investigational new drug (IND) study. The main objective is to establish quickly whether the agent is at all working in human recipients or not. Thus, it will eliminate the ineffective or unwanted materials from the study. Preclinical requirements are reduced and exposure to patient becomes very minimal. It requires also only 4-12 participants in a single centre cohort and usually completed in less than one-month time.

Features of Phase 0
- Only a few numbers of volunteers are involved.
- Micro dose is given, almost <1% of therapeutic dose.
- Operational aspects, ethical procedures similar to conventional trial
- Strict regulatory monitoring or GCP principles are not required
- Dose escalation may be allowed in some cases
- It does not have any therapeutic intent
- Not intended to study drug tolerance/ safety features
- Provides preliminary information regarding mechanism of action, pharmacokinetic and pharmacodynamic features.

Phases of Clinical Trial

Clinical trial is the research which studies new tests and treatments and evaluate their effects on human outcomes. People are recruited voluntarily to take part in different phases of trial to evaluate medical interventions including drugs, cells and other biological products, surgical procedures, radiological procedures, devices, behavioral treatments and preventive care. All clinical trials are very carefully planned, designed. Clinical trial consists of 4 phases.

Phase I (Safety and Dosage): Done by clinical pharmacologists
Subject: 20 – 25 human healthy volunteers / may be patients
Type: Non-blind / open studies, Randomization

Objectives
- Maximum tolerated dose
- PK parameter & PD parameter
- Dose range, safety profile and tolerability (Data obtained are utilized in phase II)

Phase II (Efficacy and Side Effects):
Done by clinical pharmacologist

Subject: Early phase – 20 – 200, Late phase – 50 – 300
Objective: Efficacy, Dose range and Final dosage

Phase III (Efficacy and Monitoring of ADR)
Done by clinician.
Subject: Patients, several hundred to several thousand.
Type: Multicentric, randomized, blinded, placebo controlled.
Objective:
- Further safety and efficacy in wide range of population
- Confirm information gathered in Phase I, II.
- Used in different stages of disease
- Drug -drug interaction noted.

At the end statistical calculation done e.g., t-test, chi square test, ANOVA and others for statistical significance, confidence limit is set. Both the safety efficacy is evaluated. After completion of this phase, manufacturer. Company can apply to the regulatory authority for marketing approval of drug.

Phase IV: (Post Marketing Study/ Safety and Efficacy)
Done by clinician where subjects are patients
Objectives
- Ensuring safety and efficacy in different ethnic gr.
- Monitoring a drug's long-term effect.
- Drug interaction and newer indications detected.
- Impact on patient quality of life.
- Cost effectiveness
- Comparison of a drug with other drugs already in market.
- Remaining several years as new drug status

Section 2: Important terms

Blinding and Allocation Concealment

Allocation Concealment	Blinding
Sequence of randomization is concealed	Intervention is not known to subjects/investigator /both
Usually guards selection bias	Observation bias is prevented
Occurs during recruitment	After recruitment

Control Group

In scientific experiments, control group is the group of subjects that receives no treatment or a standardized treatment. Control groups have no outcome of interest at the time of selection. Using control group, we can say that any observed effects in research may be due to the treatment effect. Control group acts as a point of reference against which outcome is judged.

Types

They are sampled independent of exposure status which means that probability of selection of exposed and unexposed control is equal. Control is best recruited from the population which produced cases.

Types- Placebo Control, Dose-Comparison Concurrent Control, No Treatment Concurrent Control, Active Treatment Concurrent Control, Historical Control.

Ethical Issues
- ❖ Participant must be informed about receiving or not receiving the actual treatment
- ❖ Using placebo when effective treatment is available is serious ethical concern

What Happens if There is No Control Group?
- ❖ Without a control group, it is difficult whether responses are due to the treatment or have occurred naturally
- ❖ Confounding effect cannot be ruled out
- ❖ There may be risk of bias in the result
- ❖ Reliability and validity of the study become challenging

Surrogate Endpoint

It is a measure of certain treatment that may correlate with a real endpoint but does not have a guaranteed relationship. Before a surrogate endpoint can be accepted, evidence from epidemiological studies and clinical trials are required. Surrogate endpoints that have undergone extensive testing (validated) are accepted by the FDA. FDA's surrogate endpoint table provides valuable information for drug developers.

Applications
- The outcomes take a very long time to develop
- Where the real end points correlate well with the surrogate endpoints and is well understood
- Studying clinical endpoint would be unethical (e.g. mortality in heart disease)
- The use of surrogate endpoints in clinical trials may allow earlier approval of new drugs to treat serious or life-threatening diseases, such as cancer.

CD4 count is a surrogate marker for death from HIV infection. Cholesterol is a surrogate marker of heart disease. Death from heart disease is the real end point of interest but here cholesterol is taken as marker. Fragmented blood cells may be surrogate marker for organ failure. In many cases when studies using surrogate markers showed benefit from a particular treatment but later, repeat study aimed at real endpoint showed no benefit, or even harm. Sometimes it is difficult to interpret a study which uses surrogate marker as primary measure of outcome. Adequate validation is required before using it as a surrogate marker. Approval of drug product on the basis of benefit using surrogate marker may pose a legal problem. Accelerated approval of drugs has been criticized by many in the scientific community.

Pilot Study

Pilot study is a small study to test research protocols, data collection instruments, sample recruitment strategies, and other research techniques in preparation for a larger study. For conducting a good research study and to obtain a high-quality valid outcome, each step of research protocol has to be perfectly planned, designed. Pilot study actually is the first step which precedes the main large trial or study to foresee its feasibility and validity. Researchers get fully aware of each step of original projects during conducting the small-scale pilot study.

Types of Pilot Study
- ❖ External: Independent of original project, done separately
- ❖ Internal: Included in the design of the main study and results are also taken into consideration.

Objectives
1. To assess the feasibility of main study protocol: Pilot study follows each step same as the main study starting from inclusion, exclusion criteria; storage, testing and distribution of intervention agents; methods of data collection and analysis. Thus, researcher comes to know the loopholes or strength of the protocol.
2. Assessment of subject recruitment: Sample size estimation, rate of subject recruitment, appropriateness of consent form, consent taking process – all these can be assessed through it.
3. Randomization and Blinding assessment: Can assess if the procedure of randomization and blinding properly executed.
4. Acceptability of intervention: In a clinical trial, different groups are allocated with different intervention substances. Whatever may be the outcome, the drugs or methods may not be acceptable or suitable to some participants. A pilot study can anticipate it and give chance for rectification.
5. Selection of outcome measure: Pilot study helps to identify the appropriate primary and secondary outcome among the numbers of possible outcomes, which can best reflect the intention of researchers and keep merit in the study.
6. Data entry and analysis assessment: Steps of data entry, using of suitable software, methods of analysis, proper coding of variable can be easily assessed beforehand.

Researchers usually intend to include the data of pilot study in the main study as it may reduce the sample size, duration of study. But it is only allowed in case of internal pilot study where it included in main study procedure and planned during study designing.

Analysis

Pilot studies are not done for hypothesis testing. Usually, sample size remains very small in pilot study in comparison to original project. Therefore, though full analysis of pilot study data has to be done, but result does not influence the occurrence of main study whether it becomes statistically significant or insignificant.

Fate of Main Study after Pilot Study

Main study may be terminated
Proceed with main study after modification of study design
Proceed with main study without modification of design
Thorough monitoring not modification required.

Randomization

Results of research should reflect the true treatment effect. In order to do that, we are to guard against biases. Randomization procedure is used in clinical trial and many biological experiments. Here each subject has equal chance of receiving any treatment under study. It prevents the selection bias and produces comparable groups in relation to known and unknown variable at the baseline. Through randomization we can eliminate bias in treatment assignments. Finally, it permits the use of probability theory and provides an unbiased estimate. Here, we get subjects in different treatment group with equal probability.

Subjects/treatments are assigned random number obtained from random number table or computer-generated random number. Effects of covariates are balanced through this method. Other than randomization, various methods to control confounding are used such as stratification, multivariate regression. In large sample size with difficult situations, we take the help of computer programming.

Common methods of randomization include simple randomization, blocked randomization, stratified randomization. Simple randomization procedure ensures randomness of assignment of subject to a particular group. Very simple procedure but in small sample, it may produce unequal sample size. In block randomization, block size is determined first which has predetermined groups having equal number of subjects. Block size should be multiple of number of treatment groups. Failure to control covariates may lead to false interpretation of treatment effect. Stratified randomization method control covariates at the base level and make groups comparable. Stratification is done for each suspected variable as for example, different age group, and sex wise classification and as per co morbidity status. Difficult to follow this procedure in case of small sample size with multiple strata.

Through online procedure, other than random number table or computer-generated random number, we can randomize subjects in clinical/biological experiments. Two online software are http://www.randomization.com, http://www.graphpad.com/quickcalcs. In GraphPad, as the seed point of local computer clock is not displayed, same randomization plan cannot be generated. With this software, 10 treatment allocations are possible. Seed number can be obtained in former software, so we can reproduce a treatment plan. In contrast to graph pad, 20 treatment assignments are possible.

Section 3: Conducting Different Types of Study

Two major steps: Ethics committee approval then Conducting Study

Steps of Ethics Committee Approval

Step 1: Identify area of research
Step 2: Frame Research question (Descriptive/Analytical) [FINER]
Step 3: Translate Research question into Objective (SMART)
Step 4: Also, state research hypothesis for analytical question
Step 5: Literature search (Identify known and unknown area)
Step 6: Prepare details of materials and methods
Step 7: Draft a protocol along with annexes and instruments
Steps 8: Seek Ethics committee approval
Step 9: Conduct study after IEC approval

Conducting Interventional Study

Step 1: Define target population and study population
Step 2: Specify study variables and scales of measurements
Step 3: Sample size calculation (specify α, β and effect size)
Step 4: Decide sampling method
Step 5: Selection criteria (Inclusion, exclusion, and source)
Step 6: Informed consent
Step 7: Randomization (care of concealment of allocation)
Step 8: Allocation in treatment groups
Step 9: Introducing intervention (also control or placebo)
Step 10: Ensure blinding
Step 11: Possible measures of preventing bias
Step 12: Specify measurement procedure
Step 13: Follow up and interim data analysis
Step 14: Reporting any ADR and manage serious ADR
Step 15: Data collection
Step 16: Data analysis

Biostatistics in Health Research

Conducting Observational Study

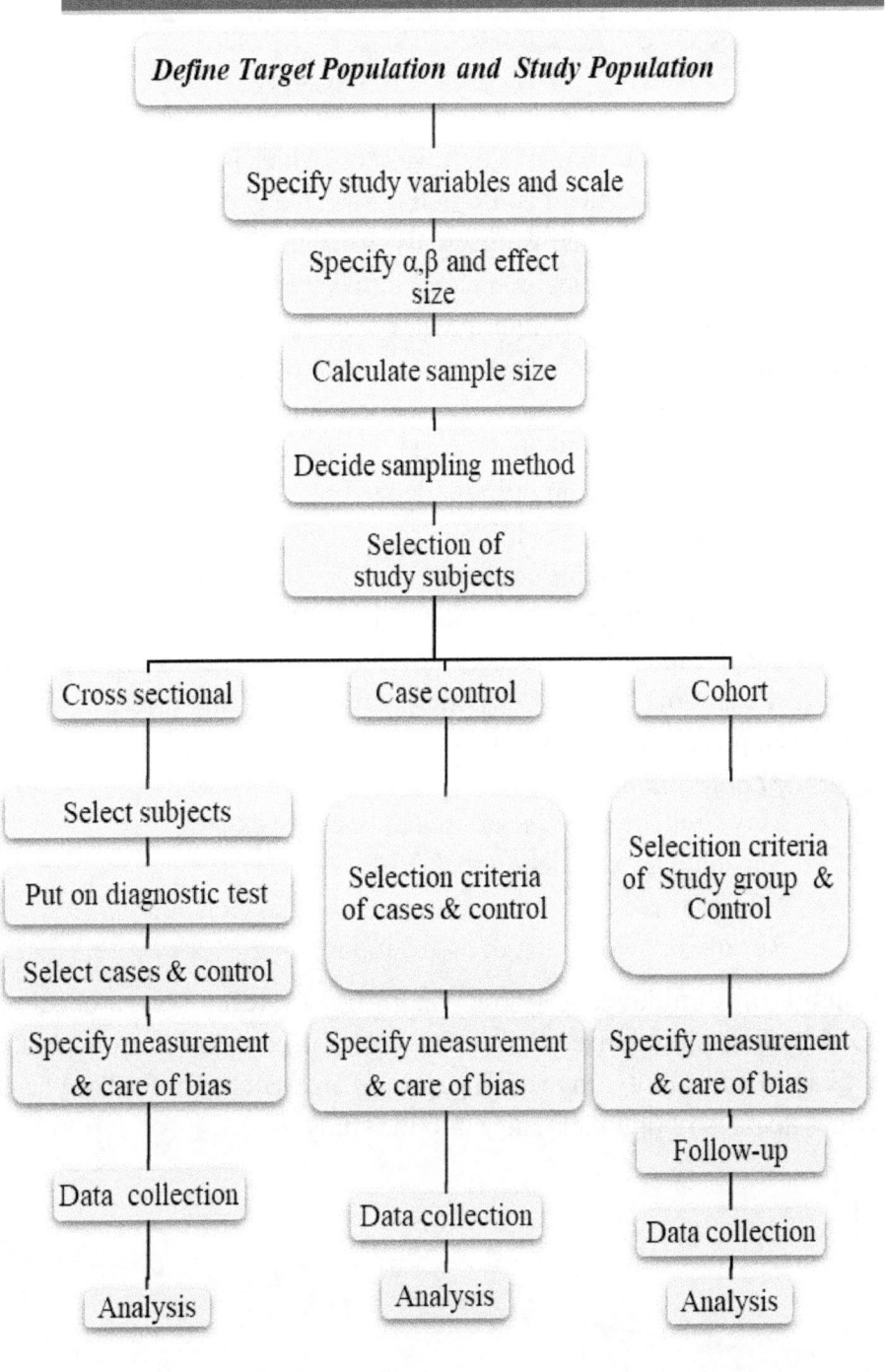

Define Target Population and Study Population

↓

Specify study variables and scale

↓

Specify α, β and effect size

↓

Calculate sample size

↓

Decide sampling method

↓

Selection of study subjects

↓

Cross sectional
- Select subjects
- Put on diagnostic test
- Select cases & control
- Specify measurement & care of bias
- Data collection
- Analysis

Case control
- Selection criteria of cases & control
- Specify measurement & care of bias
- Data collection
- Analysis

Cohort
- Selection criteria of Study group & Control
- Specify measurement & care of bias
- Follow-up
- Data collection
- Analysis

Section 4: Confounding in Research

Concept of Confounding

Sometime the effect of exposure / risk factor on outcome variable is distorted due to association of a third variable which is not relevant under study. This third variable or confounding variable is associated with both exposure and outcome and is unequally distributed within exposure and non-exposure groups being compared in the study. A confounder is not in the causal pathway as an intermediate step from exposure to outcome. As an example, if we want to measure association between obesity and coronary artery disease, age may be confounding factor which is associated with obesity and CAD both. When effect of risk factor/exposure on outcome differs depending on the level of the third variable known as effect modifier.

Magnitude of confounding is the percentage difference between crude and adjusted measures. This should be 10% or more in case of confounding. Adjusted measure of risk is computed from Mantel-Haenszel equation. Steps of detecting confounding and effect modifier have been presented in Flow Chart.

Effect of Confounding
- May simulate an association that does not exist
- May hide an association that exists
- May increase or decrease the strength of association
- Reverses the direction of association

Control of Confounding (Flow Chart 6): In restriction procedure, confounding is minimized by keeping the subjects homogeneous, but it limits generalizability. In matching, groups are matched at the base level rather than restricting their entry into the study.

Biostatistics in Health Research

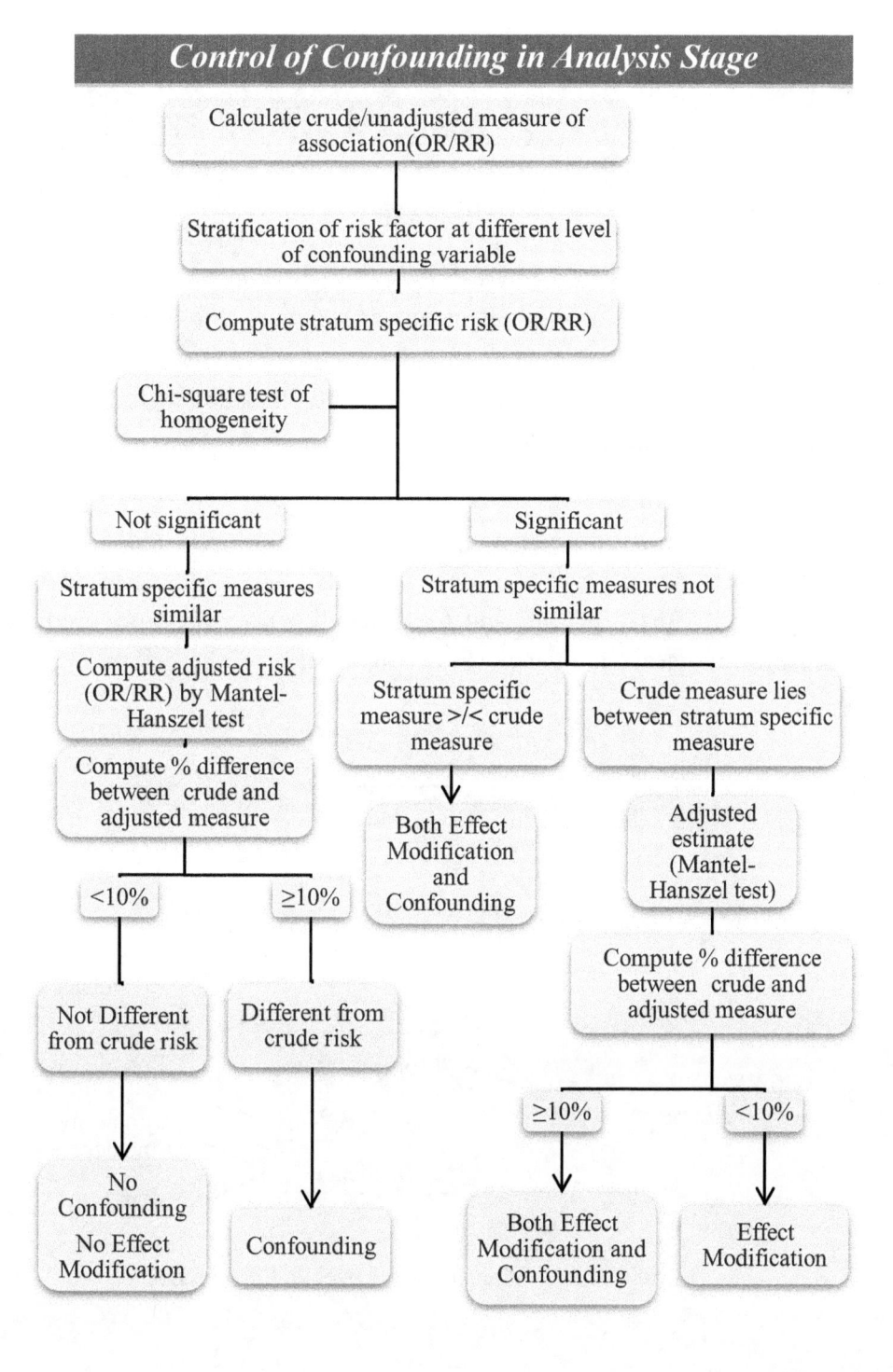

Control of Confounding in Analysis Stage

Calculate crude/unadjusted measure of association (OR/RR)

↓

Stratification of risk factor at different level of confounding variable

↓

Compute stratum specific risk (OR/RR)

↓

Chi-square test of homogeneity

Not significant → Stratum specific measures similar
- Compute adjusted risk (OR/RR) by Mantel-Hanszel test
- Compute % difference between crude and adjusted measure
  - **<10%** → Not Different from crude risk → No Confounding, No Effect Modification
  - **≥10%** → Different from crude risk → Confounding

Significant → Stratum specific measures not similar
- Stratum specific measure >/< crude measure → Both Effect Modification and Confounding
- Crude measure lies between stratum specific measure → Adjusted estimate (Mantel-Hanszel test) → Compute % difference between crude and adjusted measure
  - **≥10%** → Both Effect Modification and Confounding
  - **<10%** → Effect Modification

Chapter 5: Measures of Health Outcome

Section 1: Measures of Disease Frequency

Basic Terms

Before going to discussion proper, I want to point out three basic measures of frequency. These three are the. These include

Ratio: Where numerator is not included in denominator such as Male Female ratio.

Proportion: Where numerator is included in denominator such as proportion of males which means $\frac{Male}{(Male+Female)}$. Proportion gives idea of probability expressed as number or percentages.

Rate: It is basically a proportion, but time relationship is added. Now I shall discuss the measures of disease frequency. These are Incidence and Prevalence. Mortality Rate and Case Fatality Rate are also used as measures of disease frequency (Flow Chart 1&2).

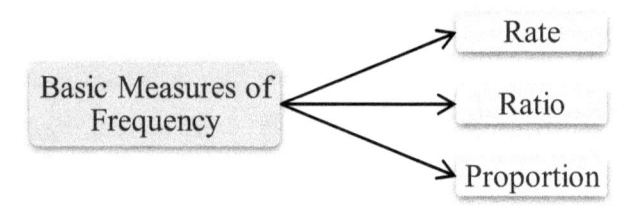

Flow Chart 1: Basic Measures of Disease Frequency

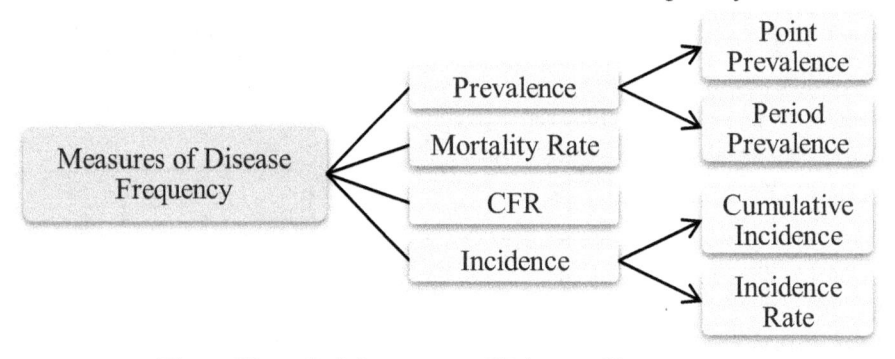

Flow Chart 2: Measures of Disease Frequency

Prevalence

It is defined as the ratio of existing old and new cases in a specific time period to that of total subjects studied at that time. It is of two types: point and period prevalence. Point prevalence measures disease frequency at a given point of time whereas in period prevalence, information collected over a period. Period prevalence is a mixture of incidence and prevalence and is not useful for research purposes. It should be noted that collection of information while estimating may continue over a period, but subjects are examined once and supposed to have done at a particular time. This is very important. Table 1 shows differences between prevalence and incidence.

Application of Prevalence
- Measures burden of disease
- Assessment and planning health care services
- Study of chronic diseases

Incidence

Incidence = Number of new cases over a period of time/Population at risk at the start of study. It is of two types:

Cumulative Incidence –same definition of incidence, only point to mention here is that it is used when study is carried out for a short period and population is stable.

Incidence Density/Incidence Rate-is used when study is of long duration and population is not stable (chance of attrition problem).

$$\text{Incidence Rate} = \frac{\text{Number of new cases}}{\text{Total person time of observation}}$$

Other measures:

Case Fatality Rate (CFR) is given by the formula
= Death due to a particular disease/Total number of cases

Application of Incidence
- Trend of disease
- Evaluation of an impact of a prevention program

Whereas in mortality rate, denominator includes total population and thus it measures the burden of disease in population. Case fatality rate denotes severity of a disease. Finally remember that measurement process should possess two essential requirements which are validity and reliability. Please don't forget this message.

Table 1: Difference Between Prevalence and Incidence

Prevalence	Incidence
Numerator includes both old and new cases	Numerator includes new cases only
Denominator includes subjects studied	Denominator includes population at risk at the start
No follow up	Requires follow up
Examined only once	Examined twice or more
Temporal relationship cannot be established	Temporal relationship can be established

Risk

Risk Definition

Probability of developing an outcome in an individual exposed to factor/s that might be but not necessarily responsible for that outcome. By the term risk, we simply mean proportion of the individual developing an outcome. For a particular outcome, population proportion is expressed by means of CI and is given by CI for proportion = $p \pm Z \times \sqrt{\frac{p \times q}{n}}$. But the main disadvantage is that it is restricted to single population. For better assessment of risk, we compare it with another group such as risk in exposed versus non-exposed group.

Measures of Risk

- ❖ Odds Ratio (OR)
- ❖ Relative Risk (RR)
- ❖ Absolute Risk Reduction
- ❖ Attributable Risk
- ❖ Number Needed to Treat/Harm (NNT, NNH)

Probability, Odds and OR

Probability: It represents ratio of number of events occurring to that of total events. It is expressed as decimal form or % form.

Odds: Odds represents ratio of probability of events occurring divided by probability of events not occurring. Let us take an example. Drug A cures a disease in 50 patients out of 60 patients treated. So, probability of cure is 50/60 i.e., 0.83 or 83%. Now probability of not cure is (1-0.83) i.e., 0.17 or 17%. Thus, Odds = 0.83/0.17 = 4.8.

Odds Ratio (OR)

Now, consider again the hypothetical study on exposure and disease status and we will calculate OR from Table 1.

Table 2: Disease and Exposure Summary

Risk	Diseased	Non-diseased
Exposed	10(a)	15(b)
Non-exposed	5(c)	10(d)

Probability of disease among exposed $= \dfrac{a}{a+b} = \dfrac{10}{25}$

Probability of non-disease among exposed $= \dfrac{b}{a+b} = \dfrac{15}{25}$

So, Odd of disease among exposed $= \dfrac{a}{b} = \dfrac{10}{15}$

Probability of disease among non-exposed $= \dfrac{c}{c+d} = \dfrac{5}{15}$

Probability of non-disease among non-exposed $= \dfrac{d}{c+d} = \dfrac{10}{15}$

So, Odds of disease among non-exposed $= \dfrac{c}{d} = \dfrac{5}{10}$

Thus, OR $= \dfrac{(10 \times 10)}{(15 \times 5)} = 1.33$ (Table 2)

CI of OR

The odds of disease with exposure are 1.33 times greater than the odds of disease in non-exposed. Now is it significant? For this, we will have to calculate confidence interval of Odds ratio. If interval includes 1, then it is not significant. Steps of calculation of CI is described below. We want to calculate 95% CI, so Z is 1.96. 95% CI for odds ratio:

$$CI = e^{Ln(OR) \pm Z\sqrt{\frac{1}{a}+\frac{1}{b}+\frac{1}{c}+\frac{1}{d}}} = e^{Ln(4) \pm 1.96\sqrt{\frac{1}{10}+\frac{1}{5}+\frac{1}{5}+\frac{1}{10}}}$$

After calculation, we get the interval (1.14-18.26) and we are 95% confident that true OR lies within this interval. As it does not include 1, effect is significant. OR requires two variables, one is outcome variable (binary in nature) and other is predictor variable which is either categorical or continuous. We have described above OR calculation when predictor is categorical (binary) but calculation of the same for continuous predictor involves complex mathematical procedure. OR is calculated in case control, cross sectional and cohort study. We frequently encounter in case of logistic regression where predictors contribution is stated in terms of OR.

Interpretation of OR

Value ranges between 0 to infinity

$OR = 1$	*Exposure is not associated with outcome*
$Log\ OR = 0$	*Exposure is not associated with outcome*
$OR > 1$	*Exposure is positively associated*
$Log\ OR > 0$	*Exposure is positively associated*
$OR < 1$	*Exposure is negatively associated*
$Log\ OR < 0$	*Exposure is negatively associated*

Predictor is categorical: Interpreted against reference category
Predictor is continuous: Interpreted per unit change in predictor
In logistic regression, effect of predictors as a change in OR.

Problem 1: To determine the association between diabetes and hypertension, researcher selected 200 diabetic patients and 400 non diabetic patients. It was found that 50 of the diabetics and 20 of the nondiabetic subjects are hypertensive. Calculate OR and 95% CI.

Biostatistics in Health Research

Section 2: Frequently Asked Questions

1. A post graduate trainee of pharmacology that he will determine the burden of depression among 300 patients of Covid 19, he included both OPD and indoor patients. 12 patients had previous history of depression and 74 patients developed it during the study period. Find incidence of depression in the study population? *(25.7%per year)*

2. In Nischinta village of Asansol subdivision, there were 28 snake bite cases last year, 12 cases presented or confirmed cases of poisonous snake bite and were hospitalized, four of them died. Calculate the case-fatality ratio. [*= (2/28) *100=7.14% case fatality ratio in snake bite*]

3. A prospective cohort study with 3000 subjects was carried out to see the beneficial effect of exercise on coronary heart disease. 2000 people are on exercise and 1000 are not doing exercise. At the start of study all were free of coronary artery disease. They were followed up for 10 years. 30 subjects among those who are on exercise and 40 among those who are not on exercise developed coronary artery disease diagnosed by ECG. Calculate Relative risk.

4. In a community health checkup, 20 adolescents were detected having anaemia. Total number of subjects studied 140. What is the appropriate measure of disease frequency? Calculate it. *Appropriate measure is point prevalence. So as per formula, point prevalence of anaemia among adolescent girls= 20/140 = 14.29%*

5. In a community, out of 900 villagers 10 developed a disease in one-month period. It is also found that 100 people already suffered from that disease and 400 people are immunized against the disease. What is the appropriate measure of disease frequency and calculate it? [*Population at risk = 900 − (400 + 100) = 400, So, CI = 10/ 400 = 2.5%*]

6. A total of 200 people with diabetes were followed up for 4 years to observe for the development of nephropathy in a cohort study. At the end of first year, 32 people left the study, none developed nephropathy. At the end of 2nd year, one subject developed nephropathy, 18 people left the study. At the end of 3rd year, four people developed nephropathy, ten left the study. At the end of 4th year, one subject developed nephropathy. Calculate incidence rate in this study?

7. What is NNT and NNH?

NNT is used to quantify measure of effectiveness associated with an intervention whereas NNH to quantify measure of harm associated with an intervention.

Calculation

Both NNT and NNH are calculated in the same way and is given by the formula:

$$\text{NNT or NNH} = \frac{1}{Absolute\ Risk\ Reduction(ARR)}$$

Suppose, outcome of interest (Effectiveness or Harm) E_I and E_0 in treatment or exposed group and control group respectively. So, denominator ARR= E_0- E_I when calculating NNT and ARR= E_I- E_0 in case of NNH. (ARR is difference in event rates between groups)

Problem 1

If event of interest with a drug is (E_I) 40% and in control group (E_0) is 60%. Calculate NNT.

ARR=0.6-0.4 =0.2. So, NNT=1/ARR=5.

How to define?

NNT is defined as the number of patients need to be treated for one additional patient to get benefit compared to control group. NNH is defined as the number of patients need to be exposed to a risk factor/treatment for one additional patient to experience harm compared to control group.

Interpretation

NNT 5 means 5 patients need to be treated to have beneficial effect/response to therapy in one additional patient. Similarly, NNH 60 means 60 patients need to be exposed or treated to have one adverse effect of treatment or risk factor.

Chapter 6: Statistical Tests

Section 1: Statistical Procedure

Different procedures for statistical tests are shown in Flow Chart 1.

Descriptive Statistics

Describing properties of a sample or of population. In descriptive type of studies, no hypothesis testing is required; no comparisons, only measures of central tendency and measures of dispersion and correlation are described. There is no inference about population from the sample.

Domain of descriptive statistics
- Statistics of location (central tendency)
- Statistics of dispersion (spread of data)
- Relationship between two variables (Correlation)

Inferential Statistics

Drawing inference about the properties of populations from samples. It involves hypothesis testing (t-test, Chi-square test, ANOVA etc.)

Prediction Statistics

Predicting behavior from current observations e.g. Regression analysis (This will be discussed in chapter of correlation and regression).

During reporting results of a research work, descriptive part is always important whatever may be the types of study and procedure. It is presented in first part of analysis section. Averages, standard deviation/variances are the main focus. When our objective is inference or drawing conclusion about population from the sample values, hypothesis testing is necessary. For hypothesis testing, numerous statistical tests are available. Amongst those, appropriate test selection is the most vital step. Different research questions are handled through selection of appropriate test (Flow Chart 2). Then we will discuss, different tests for research questions.

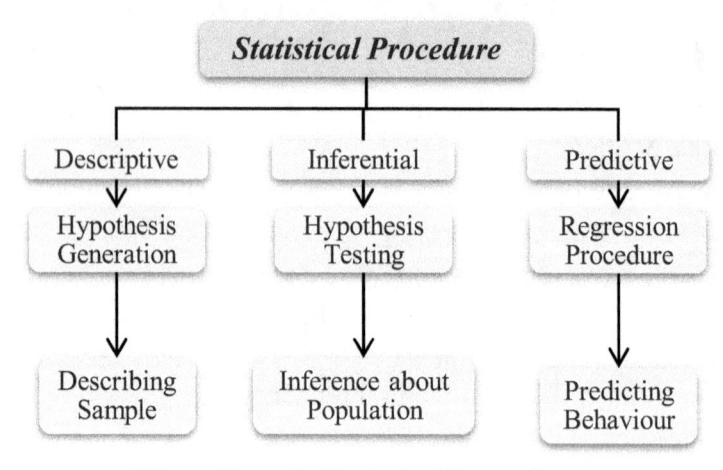

Biostatistics in Health Research

Flow Chart 1: Statistical Procedure

```
                    Statistical Procedure
          ┌──────────────┼──────────────┐
     Descriptive     Inferential     Predictive
          ↓              ↓              ↓
     Hypothesis      Hypothesis      Regression
     Generation       Testing        Procedure
          ↓              ↓              ↓
     Describing     Inference about  Predicting
      Sample         Population      Behaviour
```

Flow Chart 1: Statistical Procedure

Flow Chart 2: Research Questions

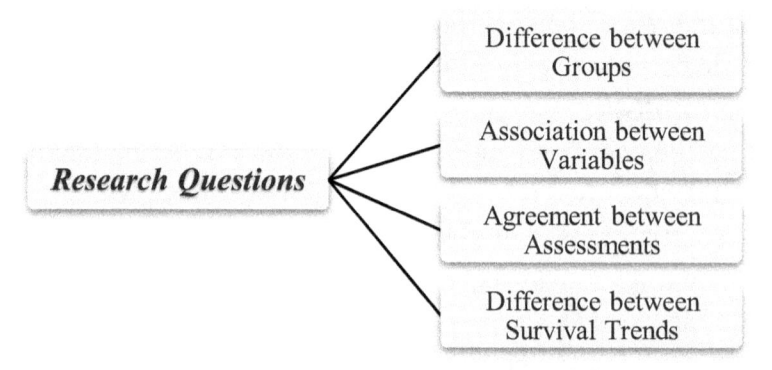

Research Questions:
- Difference between Groups
- Association between Variables
- Agreement between Assessments
- Difference between Survival Trends

Flow Chart 2: Research Questions

In this chapter, our research questions have been focused on One Sample Test (Flow Chart 3), Difference between Groups (Flow Chart 4A,4B) and Association between Groups (Flow Chart 5). Agreement Statistics and Survival Analysis have discussed in separate chapters. If overall result comes significant, multiple group comparison needed - Dunn's test, Tukey 'test and Dunnett's test.

Biostatistics in Health Research

One Sample Test

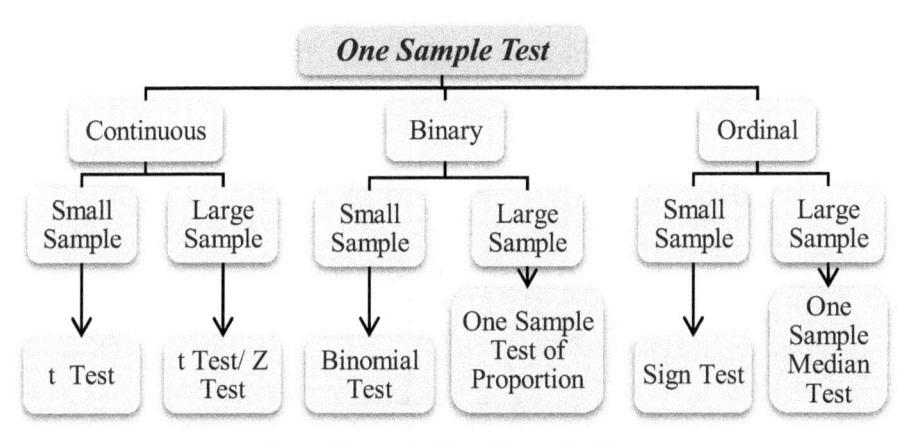

- Continuous
  - Small Sample → t Test
  - Large Sample → t Test / Z Test
- Binary
  - Small Sample → Binomial Test
  - Large Sample → One Sample Test of Proportion
- Ordinal
  - Small Sample → Sign Test
  - Large Sample → One Sample Median Test

Flow Chart 3: One Sample Test

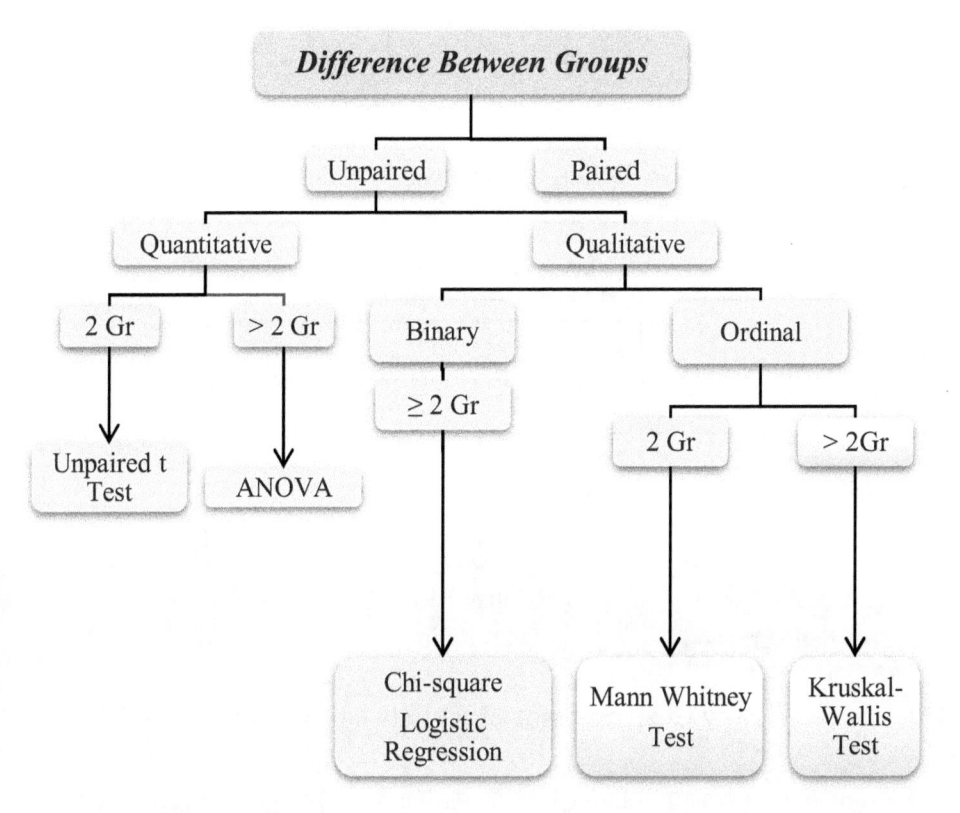

Difference Between Groups

- Unpaired
  - Quantitative
    - 2 Gr → Unpaired t Test
    - > 2 Gr → ANOVA
  - Qualitative
    - Binary
      - ≥ 2 Gr → Chi-square, Logistic Regression
    - Ordinal
      - 2 Gr → Mann Whitney Test
      - > 2 Gr → Kruskal-Wallis Test
- Paired

. Flow Chart 4A: Difference Between Groups (Unpaired)

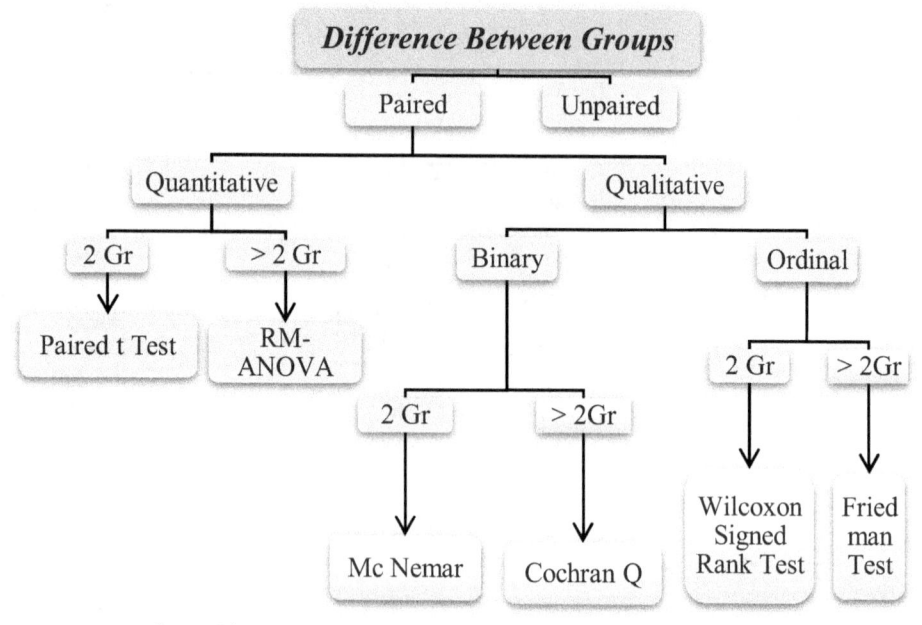

Biostatistics in Health Research

Difference Between Groups

- Paired
  - Quantitative
    - 2 Gr → Paired t Test
    - > 2 Gr → RM-ANOVA
  - Qualitative
    - Binary
      - 2 Gr → Mc Nemar
      - > 2 Gr → Cochran Q
    - Ordinal
      - 2 Gr → Wilcoxon Signed Rank Test
      - > 2 Gr → Friedman Test
- Unpaired

Flow Chart 4B: Difference Between Groups (Paired)

Association Between Variables

- Qualitative
  - > 2 Variables → χ^2 Test for Trend, Logistic Regression
  - 2 Variables → Relative Risk, Odds Ratio
- Quantitative (2 Variables) → Correlation Coefficient (r)

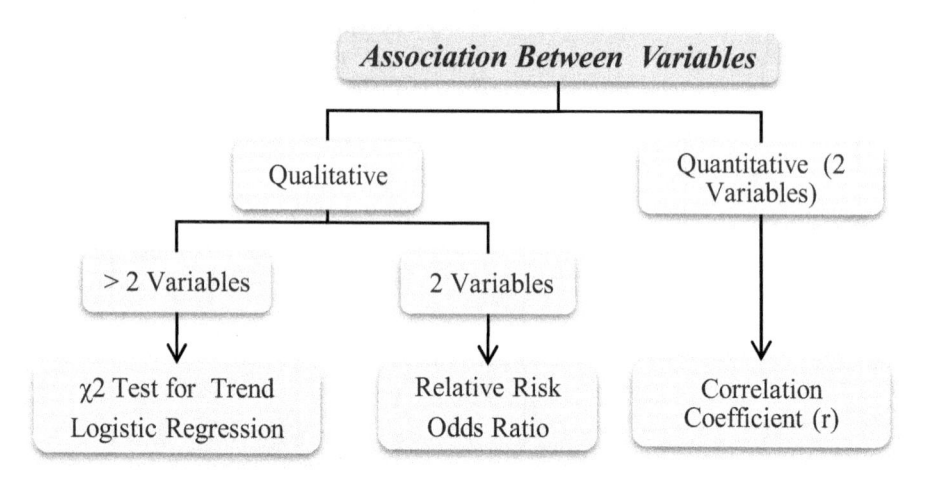

Flow Chart 5: Association Between Variables

(Source of Flow Chart 1- Flow Chart 5: Parikh MN, Hazra A, Mukherjee J, Gogtay N. Research Methodology Simplified: Every Clinician a Researcher. 1st ed. New Delhi: Jaypee Brothers Medical Publishers; 2010.)

Section 2: Assumptions of Statistical Test

Usually, three assumptions are tested before carrying out common statistical tests. These are Normal Distribution, Homogeneity of Variances and there should be no outlier.

Measures of Normal Distribution

Normality assumption is checked in t test, ANOVA, Correlation and Regression analysis. Various methods are described below.

Skewness-In a normal distribution skewness is zero and is given by the formula $S = \left[\frac{(X-\bar{X})}{SD}\right]^3$

Kurtosis- represents peak ness of a given distribution and is given by $K = \left[\frac{(X-\bar{X})}{SD}\right]^4$, In a normal distribution, Kurtosis should be zero.

Tests for Normality
- Anderson-Darling test
- Ryan –Joiner normality test
- Shapiro-Wilk Test-Measures correlation between data and corresponding normal score and is commonly used test. It is useful in small sample size.
- Kolmogorov-Smirnov test

Solution for non-normal distribution: Log transformation or other types of transformation and then carry out the procedure.

Homogeneity of Variances

Squared average distance of scores from their respective mean are equal across all groups. Variances are not significantly different from each other statistically.

Detection of Homogeneity of Variances
- Graphical method: Box whisker plot which depicts groups of numerical data through quartiles.
- Tests: In case of two groups-F test, When more than two groups- Levene's test and Bartlett's test

F Test

F test and ANOVA both uses F statistic. F test compares variances between groups whereas ANOVA compares multiple means.

F in F test is given by: $F = \dfrac{Variances\ of\ Group\ 1}{Variances\ of\ Group\ 2}$

In ANOVA, $F = \dfrac{Variability\ explained\ by\ treatments}{Variability\ not\ explained}$

Null Hypothesis: Variances of two groups are equal ($SD_1^2 = SD_2^2$)
Alternate Hypothesis: Variances are not equal
F test is usually one tailed, but may be two tailed.

This test is particularly useful in testing assumptions (equality of variances) in many statistical tests, to compare treatment variance in clinical trial, comparing variability in production process (quality control) and variability in genetic makeup.

Use Excel Function F.Test.

Problem 1: CRP conc. after antimicrobial therapy. Test the assumption whether homogeneity of variances present.

Group 1: 1, 1.5, 3, 2, 2, 2, 0.9, 2.2, 1.6, 1.5, 2.2
Group 2: 3, 2, 4, 2, 5, 8, 2, 6, 6, 2

Table 1: F Test for Comparing Variances

	Group 1	Group 2
Mean	1.8	4.2
Variance	0.395	4.2
Observations	10	10
df	9	9
F	0.094	
P(F<=f) one-tail	0.0008	
F Critical one-tail	0.314	

Levene's Test

This test is used to detect homogeneity of variances when there are more than 2 groups. Levene's test is commonly used in research analysis during assumption testing. Very easy to calculate manually. Most of the software give output of this test.

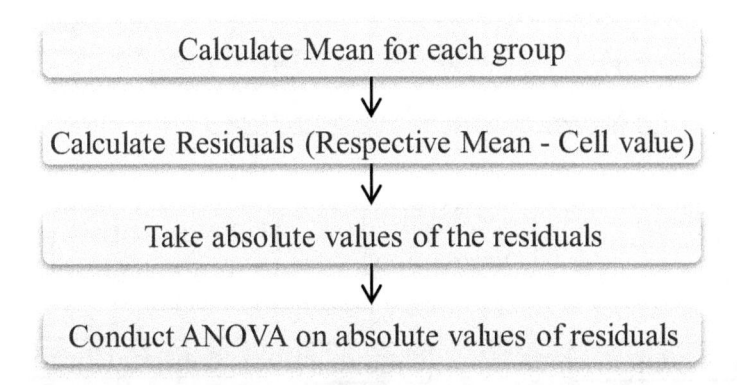

```
┌─────────────────────────────────────┐
│  Calculate Mean for each group      │
└─────────────────────────────────────┘
                  ↓
┌─────────────────────────────────────┐
│ Calculate Residuals (Respective Mean - Cell value) │
└─────────────────────────────────────┘
                  ↓
┌─────────────────────────────────────┐
│  Take absolute values of the residuals │
└─────────────────────────────────────┘
                  ↓
┌─────────────────────────────────────┐
│ Conduct ANOVA on absolute values of residuals │
└─────────────────────────────────────┘
```

Outlier

These are unusual point and lies in the extremes of dataset. They may contain useful information and that is the reason we should always remain alert of its existence. It may be related with one variable only (univariate outlier) or may be multivariate which is linked with at least two variables.

Presence of outlier may be due to typographical mistake. It may be due to measurement error. Sometimes, outliers are retained in analysis and reported in the result section. It may distort the result and bias may occur. There is false interpretation of outcome.

Detection of Outlier

- ❖ Z score- Typically Score > 3 or < 3 are considered outlier.
- ❖ Histogram
- ❖ Box-Whisker method - 2 or 3 SD away from mean.
- ❖ IQR-1.5 IQRs below the Q1 or above the Q3 in a data set.
- ❖ Scatter plot
- ❖ Mahalanobis Distance-detects outlier in multivariate data.
- ❖ Influential Point- Cook's distance is used to measure the influence of an observation in a regression model. Predicted value is estimated when all data set are present and when a particular observation is omitted. A common rule of thumb is Cook's distance $> \frac{4}{n-p-1}$ indicates influential nature of an observation in a regression model where n is number of observations and P is the number of predictors.

Biostatistics in Health Research

Assumptions of Statistical Test (Flow Chart 6)

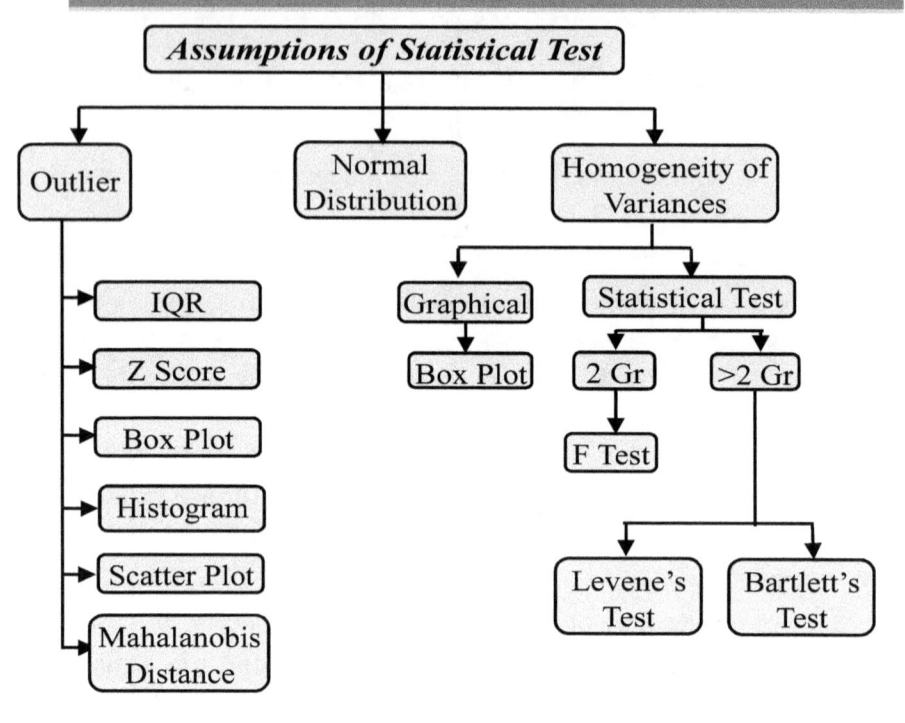

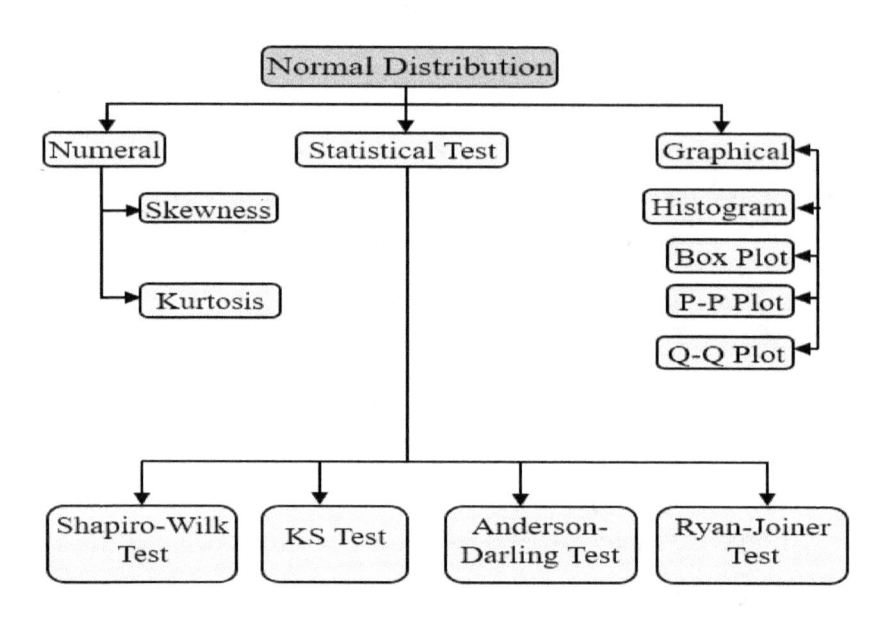

Assumptions of Statistical Test

- Outlier
  - IQR
  - Z Score
  - Box Plot
  - Histogram
  - Scatter Plot
  - Mahalanobis Distance
- Normal Distribution
- Homogeneity of Variances
  - Graphical
    - Box Plot
  - Statistical Test
    - 2 Gr
      - F Test
    - >2 Gr
      - Levene's Test
      - Bartlett's Test

Normal Distribution

- Numeral
  - Skewness
  - Kurtosis
- Statistical Test
  - Shapiro-Wilk Test
  - KS Test
  - Anderson-Darling Test
  - Ryan-Joiner Test
- Graphical
  - Histogram
  - Box Plot
  - P-P Plot
  - Q-Q Plot

Section 3: Student t Test

Basics of Student t Test

If we want to find the difference in means statistically between two groups, we carry out t-test. Data are quantitative in nature. Before going to test proper, assumptions are to be met.

Types of Student t Test (Flow Chart 6)

One Sample t Test- Group mean is compared with a hypothesized mean
Independent t-Test – Two different group mean compared (subjects are different in two group) such as BP in two groups compared
Paired Sample t-Test – Using same subjects such as BP before and after treatment.

Assumptions of One Sample t Test
- ❖ Dependent variable is continuous in nature
- ❖ Observations are independent
- ❖ Dependent variable normally distributed
- ❖ No outlier

Assumptions of Independent T test
- ❖ Dependent variable is continuous in nature
- ❖ Independent variable has two independent groups
- ❖ Normal distribution of data in all groups
- ❖ Homogeneity of variances - Squared average distance of scores from their respective mean are equal across groups. Variances are not significantly different from each other statistically. Applicable for Independent t test and ANOVA
- ❖ No outlier in any group

Assumptions of Paired t Test
- ❖ Dependent variable is continuous in nature
- ❖ Independent variable has two independent groups and are matched (Same subjects are in both groups)
- ❖ Normal distribution of measured differences
- ❖ No outlier in measured differences

Here $t = \dfrac{\overline{x_1} - \overline{x_2}}{s(\sqrt{\dfrac{1}{n_1} + \dfrac{1}{n_2}})}$ where $s = \sqrt{\dfrac{(n_1-1)s_1^2 + (n_2-1)s_2^2}{(n_1+n_2-2)}}$,

s_1 & s_2 = Standard Deviation of Sample 1 & Sample 2
n_1 & n_2 = Sample size of two groups
If t value (Calculated) is > the Table value, we reject null hypothesis.

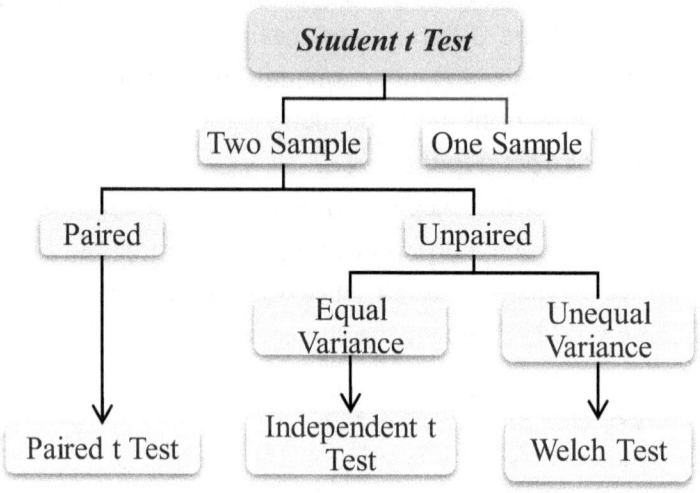

Flow Chart 6: Types of t Test

If assumptions not met, Mann-Whitney U test for Independent t test and Wilcoxon Signed Rank test for Paired test are performed. Degree of freedom(df) is important while finding table value of t. In Independent t test df = $n_1 + n_2 - 2$, in paired t test df = $n - 1$.

Z Test

Z test is done when following criteria are met:
- ❖ Standardized normal distribution
- ❖ Population variance known
- ❖ Sample size more than equal to 30

For practical purpose, we go for Z test or t test when sample size ≥ 30, and when < 30, we perform t test. When population variance or SD is known, Z test is carried out. Types of Z test and difference between Z test and t test are given below (Flow Chart 6, Table 1).

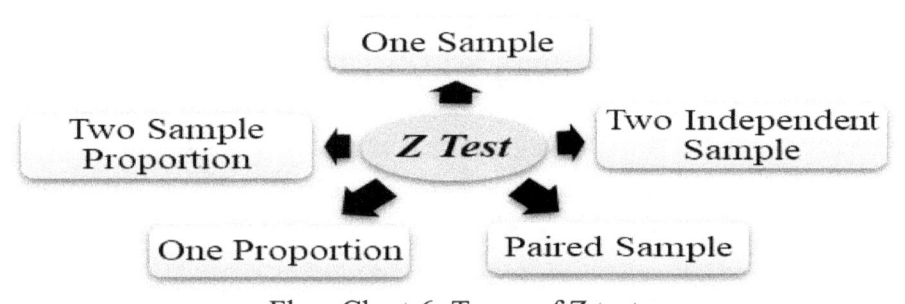

Biostatistics in Health Research

```
              ┌──────────────┐
              │  One Sample  │
              └──────────────┘
                     ▲
┌──────────────┐     │      ┌──────────────────┐
│ Two Sample   │ ◄── Z Test ──► │ Two Independent │
│ Proportion   │            │     Sample       │
└──────────────┘     │      └──────────────────┘
              ▼             ▼
    ┌──────────────┐  ┌──────────────┐
    │ One Proportion│  │ Paired Sample│
    └──────────────┘  └──────────────┘
```

Flow Chart 6: Types of Z test

Table 1: Comparison between Z Test and Student t Test

Z Test	Student t Test
Normal distribution (standardized)	t distribution
Sample size ≥ 30	Any sample size
Population SD known	Population SD not known
Degree of freedom not required	Requires degree of freedom
Can be used in test of proportion	Can not be used

Two Sample Z test for Proportion

Suppose there are two samples with a particular characteristic whose proportions are p_1 and p_2 with sample size n_1 and n_2 respectively. Z statistic is calculated as follows:

$$p = \frac{(p_1 n_1 + p_2 n_2)}{(n_1 + n_2)} \qquad Z = \frac{(p_1 - p_2)}{\sqrt{pq \times \left(\frac{1}{n_1} + \frac{1}{n_2}\right)}}$$

P=Pooled Sampled Proportion. Z table gives p value.

Z Score

In a normal distribution, location of an element can be expressed in terms of how many standard deviations it lies above or below the mean. This is the Z score. If it is above the mean, it is positive and if it below the mean, it is negative. Tables of Z scores give us the proportion of the distribution that lies above Z score. So, Z score is obtained when we divide the deviation of an element from the mean by standard deviation (Image 1). Thus, it is a transformed score of raw score and is expressed as $Z = \frac{\text{(Score of the element - Mean)}}{SD} = \frac{X - \bar{X}}{SD}$

Importance of Z Score

It tells us the probability of any randomly selected element. As Z score standardizes a distribution, it can be compared with other standardized distribution. If two scores come from two distributions, comparison is possible in two ways. Suppose a student get 70 marks in language and 58 marks in biostatistics, how it can be compared. In this situation, either mean or SD value must be known, or second method is to standardize the two distributions. Z score is calculated from the above formula and now compared between these two.

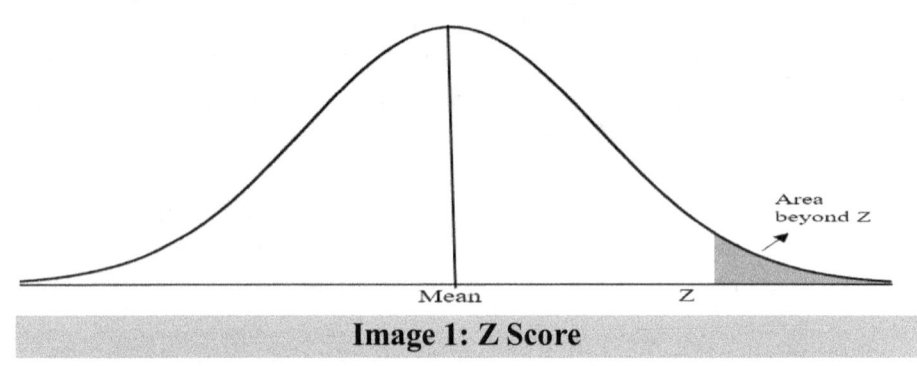

Image 1: Z Score

Degree of Freedom (df)

The term degree of freedom or simply number of independent observations or choices arises when restriction is imposed in calculation of summary measures such as mean SD and variance.

Suppose if average value of 5 observations is 15, then we are free to choose 4 observations not 5tth, because 5th value will be such that average will be 15. Similarly, in calculating SD, restrictions are imposed on 'Sum of deviations' which is zero. So, all the deviations except the last one is free to take any value. Last deviation is such which will add up to total deviation equals zero. In summary degree of freedom(df) equals one less than the sample size. Degree of freedom is important in different statistical tests where table values of t, F are found out with respect to df (from statistical table). Degree of freedom is important as it increase precision of result.

Table 2: Degree of Freedom in Common Statistical Tests

Statistical Test	Degree of Freedom
One Sample t Test	$n-1$
Independent t Tst	n_1+n_2-2
Paired t Test	$n-1$
One Way ANOVA	
Total	$n-1$
Between Groups	Number of Groups -1
Within Groups	Number of Groups -k
Chi-square Test	(Row-1) *(Col-1)

Skills on One Sample t Test

Problem: Blood pressure of ten individuals chosen from population and their blood pressure is measured. Is the sample drawn from the population of mean BP of 100 (Table 3) different?

Steps (Table 3)

Step 1: State Null and Alternate Hypothesis

H₀: Sample Mean is equal to Population Mean $H_0 : \mu = \mu_0$

H₁: This can be stated in three ways

One tailed (left)- Sample Mean < Population Mean ($H_1 : \mu < \mu_0$)

One tailed (right)- Sample Mean > Population Mean ($H_1 : \mu > \mu_0$)

Two tailed- Sample Mean(μ) ≠ Population Mean(μ_0)

Step 2: First calculate mean (Mean BP=110.6)

Step 3: $SD = \sqrt{\frac{Sum\ of\ deviation\ square}{n-1}} = \sqrt{\frac{400.4}{9}} = 6.67$

Step 4: Calculate SEM where SEM $= \frac{SD}{\sqrt{n}} = \frac{6.67}{\sqrt{10}} = 3.16$

Step 5: Calculate t value where $= \frac{(110.6-100)}{3.16} = 5.025$

Step 6: Find the degree of freedom (df), here 9

Step 7: Find out the table value of t at 9 df In excel, Table value is obtained using T.INV.2T (P value, df) for two tailed test.

Step 8: Then compare with table value of t at 9 df, α being 0.05.

Excel does not offer one sample t test. Graphpad is a free software. Type *https://www.graphpad.com/quickcalcs* then Continuous data then Analyze continuous data and then one sample t test.

Table 3: One Sample t Test

Subject	BP (systolic)	Deviation	(Deviation)^2
1	110	0.6	0.36
2	100	10.6	112.36
3	120	-9.4	88.36
4	118	-7.4	54.76
5	116	-5.4	29.16
6	114	-3.4	11.56
7	106	4.6	21.16
8	112	-1.4	1.96
9	108	2.6	6.76
10	102	8.6	73.96

Interpretation

Table value of t at 9 df =2.26, α 0.05, as calculate t value is > table value, we reject null hypothesis and conclude that sample mean is significantly different from population mean of 100. So, sample has been drawn from the different population.

Skills on Independent Sample t Test

Problem: Two groups of patients were taken to test whether their mean BP differs significantly at 5% level of significance (Table 4).

Step 1: State Null and Alternate Hypothesis
Step 2: Calculate mean of both groups
Step 3: Find the deviation in each group from their respective mean
Step 4: Square the deviation
Step 5: Add them separately in two groups
Step 6: Divide by n-1(df), df in combined sample is ($n_1+n_2 -2$)
Step 7: Calculate pooled SD where $Sp = \sqrt{\frac{(n_1-1) S_1^2 + (n_2-1) S_2^2}{(n_1+n_2-2)}}$
Step 8: Calculate t where $t = \frac{Observed\ difference\ in\ means}{S_p \left(\sqrt{\frac{1}{n_1}+\frac{1}{n_2}}\right)}$
Step 9: Find out table value of t at 18 degrees of freedom
Step 10: Compare with calculated t value. In excel, Table value obtained using T.INV.2T (P value, df) for two tailed test.

Table 4: Independent t Test

ID	Group 1	Dev 1	(Dev 1)²	Group 2	Dev 2	(Dev 2)²
1	1	0.78	0.6084	3	3	9
2	1.5	0.28	0.0784	9	-3	9
3	1.8	-0.02	0.0004	4	2	4
4	2.1	-0.32	0.1024	2	4	16
5	2	-0.22	0.0484	5	1	1
6	1.9	-0.12	0.0144	8	-2	4
7	2.2	-0.42	0.1764	10	-4	16
8	1.6	0.18	0.0324	6	0	0
9	1.5	0.28	0.0784	6	0	0
10	2.2	-0.42	0.1764	7	-1	1

Group1: Mean=1.78, $SD_1^2=0.1316$

Group 2: Mean=6, $SD_2^2=6.666$ (Table 3)

After putting all these values in the formula, $t = 15.354$, Table value of t with 18 df is 2.101 at 0.05 level, so we reject null hypothesis and conclude that two group differs with respect to BP. (*Note here that there is violation of assumption of homogeneity of variances*)

Skills on Paired Sample t Test

Problem: Ten patients were recruited for testing the effect of a drug A on BP. BP were recorded before and after administration of the drug (Table 5). Test whether there is any significant difference between before and after treatment.

Step 1: State null and alternative hypothesis (one / two tailed)

Step 2: Calculate difference in observation

Step 3: Find out mean of the difference

Step 4: Calculate $SD = \sqrt{\frac{\Sigma (Difference)^2}{(n-1)}}$

Step 5: Calculate standard error of mean $SEM = \frac{SD}{\sqrt{n}}$

Step 6: Work out t value where $t = \frac{Mean\ Differnce}{SEM}$

Step 7: Find the table value of t at 9 df, here df = n − 1 = 9

Step 8: Compare with calculated t and draw conclusion

Table 5: Paired t Test

Subject	Before treatment	After treatment	Diff	diff^2
1	142	132	10	0
2	140	136	4	36
3	150	132	18	64
4	144	140	4	36
5	140	118	22	144
6	148	134	14	16
7	152	142	10	0
8	140	136	4	36
9	150	144	6	16
10	146	138	8	4

Here, mean difference is 10 and SD 6.2. Therefore, SEM comes out to be 1.97. So, t value calculated 5.0564. From the table with 9 df, $t = 15.354$. As calculated t value is greater than table value, we reject null hypothesis and conclude that effect of drug is significant.

Welch t Test

Independent sample t test is of two types: Independent t test with equal variances and Independent t test with unequal variances. Welch t test is used when observations from two populations have unequal variances, though they follow normal distribution. Sample size may be equal or not equal in both Student t test and Welch t test. When variances are equal along with normal distribution, we calculate t as described above. Calculation of SE of difference between two means and df is different in Welch t test. There is loss of power in conducting this test if standard deviations are equal but more power when unequal. Get variance in excel typing =Var.S(). Rule of thumb is when higher to lower variance is ≥ four, we assume unequal variances. Unequal variance can be statistically tested in excel function F.TEST. We analyze in excel after installing data analysis tool kit where we get option t test with unequal variances. Significant F value says that assumptions of homogeneity of variances not met. In Table 5A, one group of neonates received Levetiracetam and other Phenobarbitone for seizure. Time to control seizure recorded, analyzed through Independent t test with unequal variances (Table 5B, Table 5C).

Table 5A: Time to Control Neonatal Seizure

Levetiracetam	Phenobarbitone
10	15
8	39
14	19
7	20
5	25
16	30
6	35
14	40

Table 5B: F-Test in Two-Sample for Variances (Excel)

	Levetiracetam	Phenobarbitone
Mean	10	27.875
Variance	17.43	91.55
Observations	8	8
df	7	7
F	0.19	
P(F<=f) one-tail	0.02	
F Critical one-tail	0.26	

Table 5C: Two-Sample t Test in Unequal Variances

	Levetiracetam	Phenobarbitone
Mean	10	27.87
Variance	17.43	91.56
Observations	8	8
Hypothesized Mean diff	0	
df	10	
t Stat	-4.84	
P(T<=t) one-tail	0.0003	
t Critical one-tail	1.81	
P(T<=t) two-tail	0.0006	
t Critical two-tail	2.23	

Section 4: Analysis of Variance (ANOVA)

Section 4.1: ANOVA

Basics of ANOVA

When we want to compare group means and number of groups is two or more, we use ANOVA, also known as analysis of variance. Here data are quantitative in nature. To reduce type I error, we avoid multiple t-test (Why?). In case of ANOVA, F value is obtained by comparing between groups variance with the within group variance and is given by: $F = \frac{\text{Between Group Variance}}{\text{Within Group Variance}}$. Between group Variance represents treatment effect whereas Within group Variance represents effect of random error. Then the calculated F value is compared with table F value with respect to df. If calculated F value > Table value, we reject null hypothesis which signifies that at least one group is different. To know which groups are significant, we perform post hoc analysis such as Tukey's test, Bonferroni test.

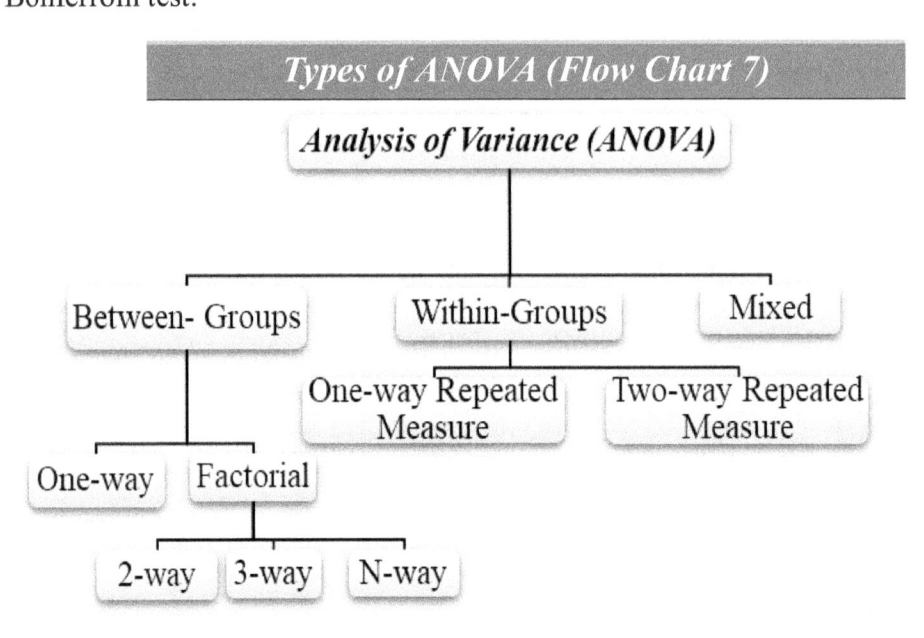

Types of ANOVA (Flow Chart 7)

Analysis of Variance (ANOVA)
- Between-Groups
  - One-way
  - Factorial
    - 2-way
    - 3-way
    - N-way
- Within-Groups
  - One-way Repeated Measure
  - Two-way Repeated Measure
- Mixed

Section 4.2: One-Way ANOVA

Basics of One-Way ANOVA

Here, there is one independent variable (IV)- quantitative that has two or more groups. In ANOVA, DV is measured in quantitative scale. Here F value (Table) depends upon degree of freedom (df) of Between Groups and Within Groups. Between-Groups / Between-Treatments represents treatment effects (explained part of variances due to intervention or variability of DV) and Within-groups/Within-treatments represents unexplained variability (random error). In all types of ANOVA, F statistic is expressed.

Hypothesis Statement

H_0: All group means are equal. H_1: At least one group mean is different

Assumptions

We should test for normal distribution, homogeneity of variance and whether outlier present or not. If assumptions are violated, Kruskal Wallis test is carried out.

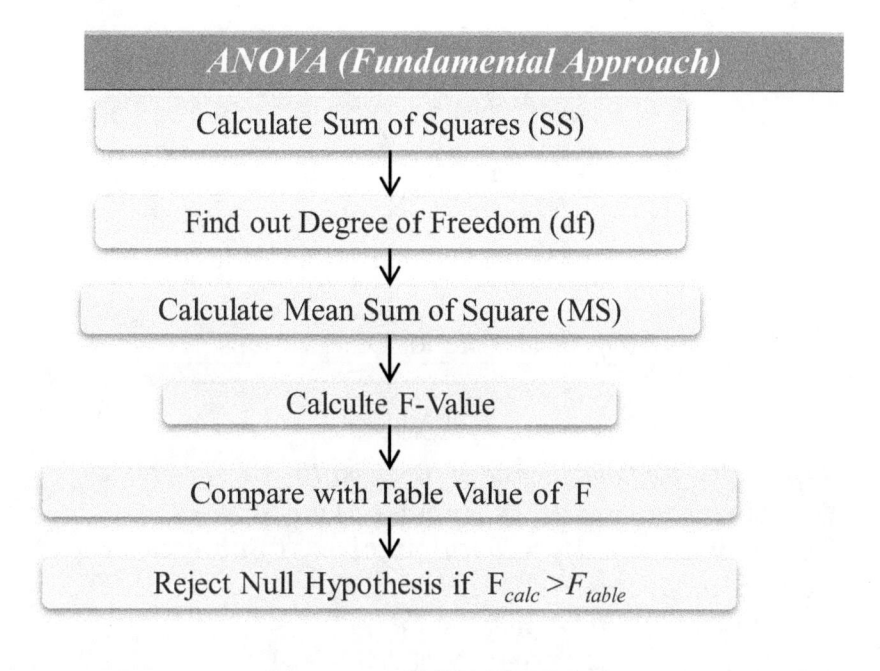

ANOVA (Fundamental Approach)

Calculate Sum of Squares (SS)
↓
Find out Degree of Freedom (df)
↓
Calculate Mean Sum of Square (MS)
↓
Calculte F-Value
↓
Compare with Table Value of F
↓
Reject Null Hypothesis if $F_{calc} > F_{table}$

Conducting One Way ANOVA (Table 6,7)

Step 1: Calculate Between-groups SS and Within-groups SS

$SS_{Between\ groups}$

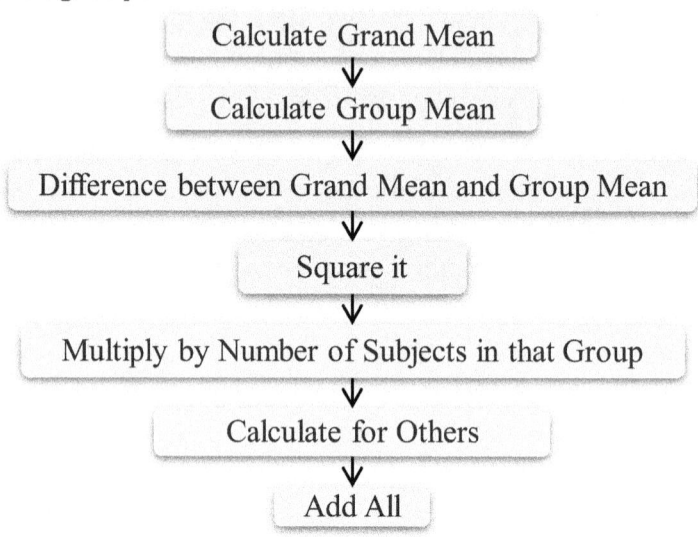

- Calculate Grand Mean
- ↓
- Calculate Group Mean
- ↓
- Difference between Grand Mean and Group Mean
- ↓
- Square it
- ↓
- Multiply by Number of Subjects in that Group
- ↓
- Calculate for Others
- ↓
- Add All

$SS_{Within\ groups}$

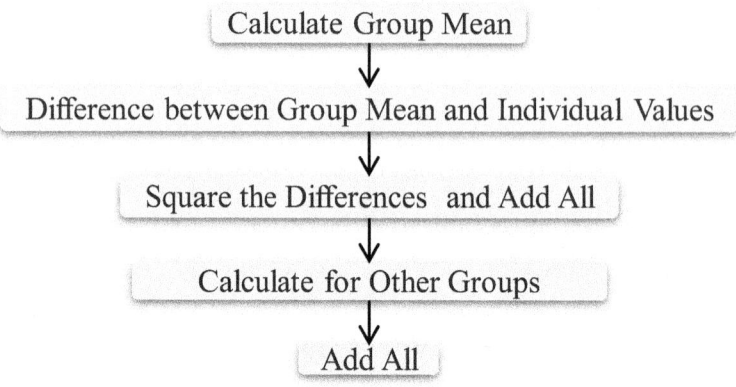

- Calculate Group Mean
- ↓
- Difference between Group Mean and Individual Values
- ↓
- Square the Differences and Add All
- ↓
- Calculate for Other Groups
- ↓
- Add All

Step 2: Now find out, degree of freedom(df)
For Between groups: $df_1 = Number\ of\ groups - 1$
For Within groups: $df_2 = Total\ number\ of\ Subjects - Number\ of\ groups$

Step 3: Calculate Mean sum square (MS)

$$MS_{Between\ groups} = \frac{SS_{Between\ groups}}{df_1}$$

$$MS_{Within\ groups} = \frac{SS_{Within\ groups}}{df_2}$$

Step 4: *Find F-value* which is given by $F = \frac{MS_{Between\ groups}}{MMS_{Within\ groups}}$

Interpretation

With df_1, df_2 and at decided level of significance, find table value of F. If calculated F > table value, reject null hypothesis.

Skills on Statistical Calculation

There are three groups: Doctors, Teachers and Farmers. Six subjects are in each group. So, it is clear that participants are different in the groups that means same participants are not involved in each group, they are different. We want to test whether their Systolic BP are different from each group or not. If differs, then to test between which groups do post hoc analysis *(Table 6,7)*.

Table 6: One-Way ANOVA

Group A	Group B	Group C
120	130	120
122	124	110
136	142	114
138	134	122
142	118	112
126	122	116

Calculate the following first then prepare analysis Table 7
Group Means and Grand Mean
$SS_{Between\ groups}$ and $SS_{Within\ groups}$
Between groups df and Within groups df
$MS_{Between\ groups}$ and $MS_{Within\ groups}$. Now calculate F

With df (2,15), Table value of F_{crit} is 3.68 and is lower than calculated value. So, we will reject null hypothesis and conclude that BP among groups differ from each other. (In excel, ANOVA: Single factor in data analysis tool kit)

Table 7: Reporting Tabe of One -Way ANOVA

Source of Variation	SS	df	MS	F	P-value	F crit
Between-Groups	781.78	2	390.89	6.40	0.009	3.68
Within- Groups	916	15	61.07			
Total	1697.7	17				

Section 4.3: Two-Way ANOVA

Basics of Two-Way ANOVA

A two-way ANOVA test is a used to determine the effect of two independent variables (IV) on a dependent variable (DV). Here IV or factor is qualitative (nominal) and dependent or outcome variable is continuous data. With this statistical technique, we can say whether variability in outcome is due to chance or due to factors. In one way ANOVA, we test the effect of one IV on DV. In three-way ANOVA, we detect the effect of three IV or factors on DV. Any ANOVA that uses more than one categorical IV is known as factorial ANOVA e.g. two-way ANOVA, three-way ANOVA. If one IV is categorical and other quantitative-Conduct ANCOVA.

Example

Three types of interventions are being given to three different groups of both sexes. We want to know whether blood pressure reduction with different types of treatment varies between male and female.

Main Purpose of Two-Way ANOVA

To test if there is any interaction between two IV on DV. But you will have to understand the meaning of the term interaction. IV has two or more levels or categories. A level is an individual category within the categorical variable. An interaction is said to be present when the effect of one IV on the DV changes depending on the level of other IV. When an interaction is significant, main effects are not interpreted in a usual way. Main effect is defined as the effect of an IV on the DV ignoring effect of other IV. Number of main effects equals number of IV. Thus, two-way ANOVA determines two things: Main effects contributed by each IV and Interaction effect between two IV on the DV.

Identifying Interaction Effect (Image 2, Table 8)

We can identify by inspection of profile plot/interaction plot. Nonparallel lines indicate interaction effect. Two drugs are being used in both sexes to evaluate mean onset time of sleep.

Table 8: Interaction Plot

Gender	Drug A	Drug B
Male	2	14
Female	16	20

We have selected two groups of subjects. Male receives Drug A and another group Female receives Drug B. Two factors are Gender and Drug group where both factors have two levels. Other than main effects of Gender and Treatment, we are able analyze to determine whether significant interaction between two factors is present or not.

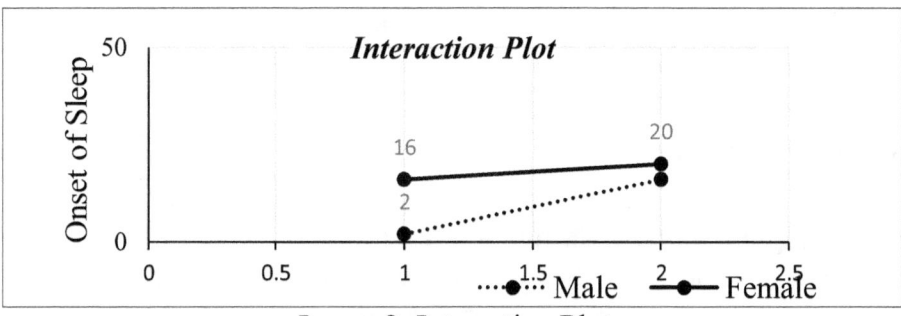

Image 2: Interaction Plot

Table 9: Two-Way ANOVA

Group	Subject	Gender	Systolic BP
Drug A	Subject 1	Male	
	Subject 2	Male	
	Subject 3	Male	
	Subject 4	Female	
	Subject 5	Female	
	Subject 6	Female	
Drug B	Subject 7	Female	
	Subject 8	Female	
	Subject 9	Female	
	Subject 10	Male	
	Subject 11	Male	
	Subject 12	Male	

Different Combinations of Effects *(Table 10)*
Table 10: Combined Effects of Factors

Effect of Factor A	Effect of Factor B	Interaction (A*B)
-	-	-
+	-	-
-	+	-
+	+	-
-	-	+
+	-	+
-	+	+
+	+	+

Principle
It uses F ratio which compares Between Group Variance with the Within Group Variance. If it is >1, there is increased likelihood that observed difference is due to IV, not due to chance.

Statement of Hypothesis
A two-way ANOVA with interaction tests three null hypotheses (Assuming there are two factors A, B):

H_O: There is no effect of factor A on DV
H_1: There is an effect of factor A on DV
H_O: There is no effect of factor B on DV
H_1: There is an effect of factor B on DV
H_O: There is no interaction between two factors
H_1: There is significant interaction between two factors

Types of Two-Way ANOVA Model
There are three types. Mainly concerned with fixed effects model.
- ❖ Fixed-Effects Model: Here levels of all the factors in the experiment are decided by the researcher, and the inferences drawn are for those specific levels.
- ❖ Random-Effects Model: Here levels of all the factors in the experiment are chosen randomly and inferences made to all possible levels, not just the ones that happened to be chosen.
- ❖ Mixed-Effects Model: This model has both fixed-effects and random-effects terms and is common.

These distinctions are important because the test statistics used to test hypotheses in the random and mixed effects models are different from the test statistics F used in the fixed effects model. Commonly we conduct two-way ANOVA assuming fixed effect model, but it is not appropriate in all situations.

Assumptions of Two-way ANOVA
- There should be two IV (categorical) one DV (continuous)
- Independence of observations-No participant should be in more than one group.
- There should be no significant outliers
- DV should be normally distributed for each combination of the levels of IV-Shapiro-Wilk test
- Homogeneity of variances for each combination of levels of IV

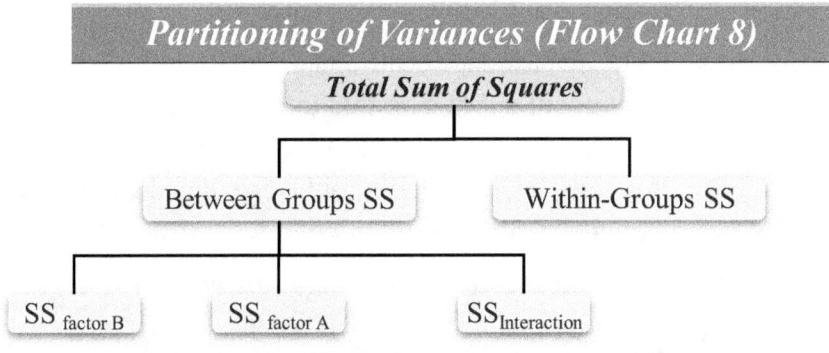

Partitioning of Variances (Flow Chart 8)

Total Sum of Squares
├── Between Groups SS
│   ├── SS factor B
│   ├── SS factor A
│   └── SS Interaction
└── Within-Groups SS

Flow Chart 8: Variances in Two-Way ANOVA

Conducting Two-Way ANOVA (Table 11)

Calculate Sum of Squares (SS)
Total SS (SS_{total})-Subtract each observation from grand average, square and then add SS for Factors (SS_A, SS_B)
Step 1: Suppose two factors A, B. A has 3 levels and B has 4 levels
Step 2: Take average of each level of each factor
Step 3: Take averages of all these averages of each factor (average of averages in any of the factors gives same grand mean).
Step 4: Subtract each average of each level of a factor from grand mean and multiply by number of observations and then add.
Step 5: In same way, find out SS for another factor.

SS_{error} -Subtract each observation from their respective level average, square it and add it and do it for all levels for the two factors and then add all

$SS_{interaction} = SS_{total} - (SS_A + SS_B + SS_{error})$

Calculate Degree of freedom (df)

$df_{total} = Total\ number\ of\ observations - 1$

df for factors:

$df_A = Number\ of\ levels - 1 = 3 - 1 = 2$

$df_B = Number\ of\ levels - 1 = 3$

$df_{interaction} = df_A \times df_B = 2 \times 3 = 6$

$df_{error} = df_{total} - (df_A + df_B + df_{interaction})$

Error df should be at least one because in calculating MSS, error df is in denominator. So, it will not be possible to calculate. Again, error mean sum of squares is in denominator and is required to calculate F value. When error df is zero, interaction cannot be calculated and interaction is said to be confounded with error term

Calculate Mean sum of squares (MS) and is given by $MS = \frac{SS}{df}$

$MS_A = \frac{SS_A}{df_A}, MS_B = \frac{SS_B}{df_B}$

$MS_{interaction} = \frac{SS_{interaction}}{df_{interaction}}, MS_{error} = \frac{SS_{error}}{df_{error}}$

Calculate F value

Fixed Effect Model:

$F_{factor} = \frac{MS\ for\ factors}{MS_{error}}$

$F_{interaction} = \frac{MS_{interaction}}{MS_{error}}$

Random / Mixed Effect Model:

$F_{factor} = \frac{MS\ for\ factors}{MS_{interaction}}$

$F_{interaction} = \frac{MS_{interaction}}{MS_{error}}$

Find the F value from table

Fixed Effect Model

> ➢ F value for factor from table (df for factor and df_{error})
> ➢ F value of interaction from table ($df_{interaction}$, df_{error})

Random Effect Model or Mixed Effect Model
- F value factor from table (df for factor and $df_{interaction}$).
- F value for interaction term is same as fixed effect model

Table 11: Two- Way ANOVA Table in Different Models

	SS	df	MS	F (fixed)	F (random/ mixed)	Table F (fixed)	Table F (mixed / random)
Factor A							
Factor B							
A*B							
Error							
Total							

Interpretation
If calculated F value is greater than table value, null hypothesis of effect due to random error or due to chance is rejected and alternate hypothesis is accepted. Mean value of each factor in a particular level gives us an estimate of effect compared to others. What we have discussed so far is the fundamental approach. We can easily do it in Excel. Many researchers take the help of statistical software. However, results are same in both the cases.

Skills on Statistical Calculation (Table 12-14)

Table 12A: Reduction of Viral Load with Anti-viral Drugs

	Male	*Female*
Drug A	5	10
	2	8
	5	4
	1	11
	3	15
Drug B	15	5
	20	18
	10	15
	25	10
	5	20

Biostatistics in Health Research

Table 12B: Two-Way ANOVA (Basic Calculation)

Mean drug A	6.4	Mean drug B	14.3
Mean male	9.1	Mean female	11.6
Grand mean	10.35		
SS total	896.55		
SS between groups	419.35		
SS drug	312.05	MS drug	312.05
SS gender	31.25	MS gender	31.25
Interaction	76.05	MS interaction	76.05
SS within groups	477.2	MS error	29.825

Here, df_{total}-19, df between groups-3, df_{drug}-1, df_{gender}-1, df interaction-1, df within groups-16.

Table 13: Group Analysis in Two-Way ANOVA

	Drug A_M	Drug A_F	Drug B_M	Drug B_F
	5	10	15	5
	2	8	20	18
	5	4	10	15
	1	11	25	10
	3	15	5	20
Group means	3.2	9.6	15	13.6
SS between	419.4			
SS within	477.2			

Table 14: Reporting Table of Two-Way ANOVA

Source of Variation	SS	df	MS	F	P-value	F crit
Drug	312	1	312.05	10.46	0.01	4.49
Gender	31.2	1	31.25	1.05	0.32	4.49
Interaction	76	1	76.05	2.55	0.13	4.49
Within/error	477	16	29.83			
Total	896	19				

From Table 14, effect of Antiviral drugs is significant in reducing viral load. Gender has no effect. Viral load reduction depends on drug therapy but not on which group participant is. This means that no interaction effect between drug and gender exists.

Section 4.4: Repeated Measures ANOVA

Basics of Repeated Measures ANOVA

The repeated measures ANOVA is used to determine whether there are any statistically significant differences between population means of three or more related groups. The groups contain same participants. Results are obtained on same dependent variable. If it includes covariate, it is known as Repeated measures ANCOVA.

Uses
- ❖ Determine if there are differences between conditions: Same dependent variable is being measured on same participants under three different conditions or managements or interventions. To analyse any significant difference in three types of managements in the treatment of anxiety (Table 15).
- ❖ Determine if there are differences between three or more time points: Same dependent variable is measured at three time points on same participants. Testing serum cholesterol conc. at three time points using newer cholesterol lowering agent and to test if there is any significant difference in measurements in different time points (Table 16).
- ❖ Determine if there are differences in change of scores: Three different conditions are being tested on same participants. Measurements are being taken at the beginning and at the end on the same dependent variable. Difference in scores is analysed using repeated measure ANOVA

Assumptions
- ❖ Normal distribution of data in each group
- ❖ No outliers
- ❖ The variances of the differences between two groups are equal. This is known as assumption of sphericity. Mauchly's test is done to detect violation of this assumption. Help of a software needed in this situation.

After giving an antihypertensive agent X to five participants and their Cholesterol conc. is being measured on 1st week, 3rd week and after one month to test whether any statistically significant difference in mean Cholesterol conc. in these time points (Table 16).

Table 15: Repeated Measure ANOVA in Different Conditions

Participant ID	Treatment 1	Treatment 2	Treatment 3
Participant 1			
Participant 2			
Participant 3			
Participant 4			
Participant 5			

Table 16: Repeated Measure ANOVA in Different Time Periods

Participant ID	Time 1	Time 2	Time 3
Participant 1			
Participant 2			
Participant 3			
Participant 4			
Participant 5			

Partitioning of Variances (Flow Chart 9)

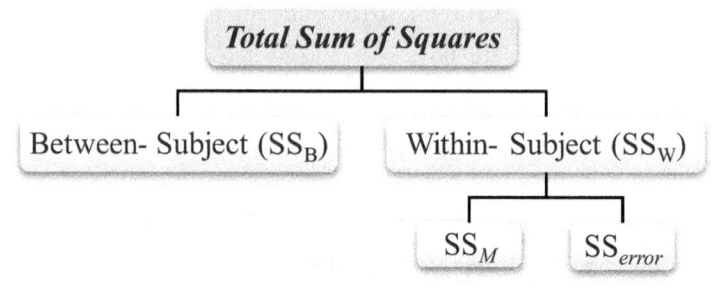

Flow Chart 9: Variances in Repeated Measure ANOVA

To calculate F value, we need to calculate different variances or sum of squares (SS). At first, we must see how the variances are partitioned (Flow Chart 9). F is calculated with the help of *SSM* and *SS error*. In excel, you may run Two factor ANOVA without replication after installing data tool kit pack. We will also calculate also Between-subjects SS(SS_B) but this is of no use for interpretation purposes.

Conducting Repeated Measures ANOVA

See Table 17-18
Step 1: Calculate Sum of Squares (SS)
At first calculate mean row wise and column wise and then grand mean (GM)
SS_{total} where $SS_{total} = \Sigma (GM - individual\ value)^2$
SS_W where $SS_W = Number\ of\ conditions \times \Sigma(cell\ value - respective\ row\ mean)^2$
SS_{model} where $SS_{model} = Number\ of\ participants \times \Sigma(GM - column\ mean)^2$. This represents treatment effects.
$SS_{error} = SS_W - SS_{model}$
Alternatively, $SS_{error} = SS_{total} - SS_B - SS_{model}$

Step 2: Find degree of freedom (df)
$df_{total} = Total\ number\ of\ observations - 1$
$df_{model} = Number\ of\ conditions - 1 (here\ 3 - 1 = 2)$
$df\ for\ Within\ subject$
$\quad\quad\quad = Total\ Observations - Number\ of\ rows$
$df_{error} = df\ for\ SS_W - df_{model} = 10$

Step 3: Find MS (Mean Sum of Square)
$MS_{model} = \frac{SS_{model}}{df_{model}}, MS_{error} = \frac{SS_{error}}{df_{error}}$

Step 4: Calculate F where $F = \frac{MS_{model}}{MS_{error}}$ *(See Table 18)*

Interpretation
Compare with table value and reject null hypothesis if it is less than calculated value of F. If the result becomes significant, in that case post hoc test such as Dunn test is to be done. F value from the Table can be obtained from excel function F.INV.RT (one tailed).

CRP conc. in three Time Periods given in table 17 to find any statistically significant difference over a period of time.

Table 17: Procedure of One- Way Repeated Measures ANOVA

Subject ID	Time 1	Time 2	Time 3	Individual mean	(Cell value-row mean) ^2
1	7	4	1	4	18.0
2	8	1	2	4	28.7
3	9	4	5	6	14.0
4	5	10	7	7	12.7
5	9	6	3	6	18.0
6	6	8	9	8	4.7
Mean CRP	7.33	6	5		96.0

Table 18: Reporting table of One- way repeated measures ANOVA

Source of Variation	SS	df	MS	F	P-Value	F crit
Between Sub	41.11	5	8.22	1.15	0.39	3.33
Within Sub	96.00	12				
Model	24.78	2	12.39	1.74	0.22	4.10
Error	71.22	10	7.12			
Total	137.1	17				

Inference
From Table 18, Model row shows, calculated F value (1.74) is less than the critical F (4.1). So, null hypothesis is retained and we conclude that Mean CRP conc. over time periods do not differ significantly. In excel, go to F.INV.RT(p value, df1, df2), putting p = 0.05, df model 2 and df error 10, it returns Fcrit 4.1.

Problem 1: Neonatologist selected 60 neonates with jaundice in a study to investigate the effect of Phototherapy. Study duration 6 days. Serum bilirubin level estimated on Day 0, Day 3 and Day 6.

Problem 2: To study the efficacy of probiotic in childhood diarrhoea, researcher took 50 patients and recorded stool frequency on Day 0, Day 2 and Day 5 after administration of ORS, Zinc and probiotic.

Section 4.5: Analysis of Covariance (ANCOVA)

Here we test if there is any difference between adjusted means in two or more unrelated group. Suppose we are measuring BP in three groups of hypertensive patients. Each group is receiving different antihypertensive drug. Group A receives drug A, Group B drug B and Group C drug C. Now if we test for difference in BP between three groups through ANOVA, there may be error. If pre-treatment BP is considered in each group, result may be different and error will be less. Here pre-treatment BP is a covariate and is a continuous variable. Hypertensive patients are IV divided into three groups. BP is DV (continuous). ANCOVA is appropriate in this situation (Table 14). Covariates are not part of the main experimental manipulation but influence the outcome. Covariates are usually continuous in nature and included in ANOVA to reduce error.

Main Purposes of Covariate in ANCOVA
- To reduce within subject variance
- To eliminate the effect of confounding

Elements of ANCOVA
- One DV- continuous in nature
- One IV with two or more levels
- One or more covariates –Continuous in nature.

Assumptions
- Residuals at each level of IV is normally distributed
- Homogeneity of variances
- Effect of covariate is independent of treatment effect.

Covariate shares variance with unexplained variance but not with treatment or manipulation part (Scenario 1 & Scenario 2). In ANOVA, total variance is divided into two parts: explained variance contributed by treatment and other is unexplained. If the treatment does not affect covariate and if we conduct ANOVA for covariate at different levels of treatment, it will be statistically not significant. This is how we can test this assumption before going to proper analysis. Remember, independence of treatment and effect of covariate is the ideal situation where we can perform ANCOVA. When covariate shares variance with treatment or explained variance, ANCOVA should not be done, otherwise there will be misinterpretation of results. This problem can be solved by randomization. Inclusion of covariate in analysis (ANCOVA), reduces unexplained variance (Scenario 2).

Scenario 1: ANOVA

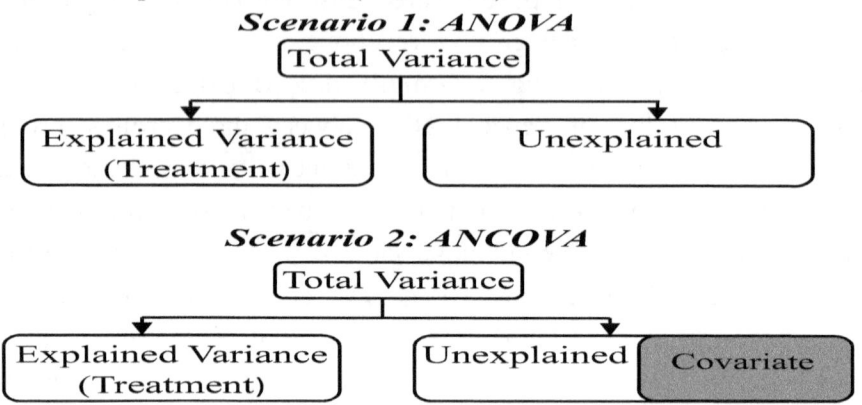

Total Variance → Explained Variance (Treatment) | Unexplained

Scenario 2: ANCOVA

Total Variance → Explained Variance (Treatment) | Unexplained | Covariate

Linear relationship between covariate and DV for each level of IV. This is verified through scatterplot and regression line at each level (Straight line). Homogeneity of regression slope is another important assumption. We assume that the relationship between the outcome (dependent variable) and the covariate is the same in each of the treatment groups. This is also tested through a scatterplot for each group of the independent variable with the covariate on one axis and the outcome on the other shows parallel lines. It is to be confirmed statistically. Image 3 shows violation of assumption as regression lines are not parallel.

Statistically, there should be no interaction between covariate and IV. In case of interaction, data transformation may help, otherwise not suitable for ANCOVA. Absence of interaction directs us to go for Analysis of Covariance (ANCOVA).

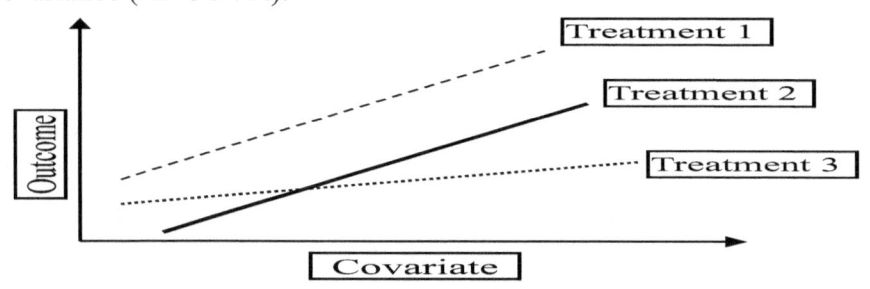

Image 3: Violation of Homogeneity of Regression Slope

Let us take an example. Five participants are in Drug A group and five participants in Drug B group (Table 19). Their body weight and systolic BP has been recorded. Does the BP differ in two groups assuming body weight may influence outcome (BP)? Use ANCOVA in this situation.

Table 19: ANCOVA

Group	Subject ID	Body Wt (Covariate)	BP (Outcome)
Drug A	1		
	2		
	3		
	4		
	5		
Drug B	6		
	7		
	8		
	9		
	10		

Example 1: Suppose an investigator is measuring BP in three groups of hypertensive patients. Each group is receiving different antihypertensive drug. Group A receives drug A, Group B receives drug B, Group C receives drug C. Now, he thought that Pre-Treatment BP and Body Weight (Continuous variable) may affect the treatment response and included in the analysis so that result may be different and error will be less. Hypertensive patients are independent variable divided into three groups. Which type of analysis? (ANCOVA)

Section 4.6: Mixed Design ANOVA

Overview of Mixed Design ANOVA

Mixed-design analysis of variance model, also known as a Split-Plot ANOVA (SPANOVA), is used to test for differences between two or more independent groups where subjects are measured over different time points. Here one factor is a fixed effects factor (between-subjects variable) and the other is a random effects factor (within-subjects variable). So, the model is a type of mixed-effects model. Advantage of this design is that we can study interaction effect of between subject factor with the within subject factor.

A researcher recruited total ten subjects and divided into two groups, one group received antihypertensive drug A and other group received drug B. Their systolic blood pressure (Table 20) is recorded in different time periods (such as week 1, week 2 and week 3). We want to know whether there is any significant interaction. Let us explain. Does the systolic BP differ in two groups over period of time? or does the systolic BP over period of time depends on which group the participants are included? or you may want to know, whether systolic BP level over different time period varies depending upon the type of intervention? In two-way repeated measure ANOVA, same subjects are followed up for different time period (Table 20).

Table 20: Mixed Design ANOVA

Group	Subject	Time 1	Time 2	Time 3
Drug A	Subject 1			
	Subject 2			
	Subject 3			
	Subject 4			
	Subject 5			
Drug B	Subject 6			
	Subject 7			
	Subject 8			
	Subject 9			
	Subject 10			

Understanding Mixed Design ANOVA

Total variation (SS_T) is partitioned into two: Between-subjects SS ($SS_{Between\ subject}$) and Within-subjects SS ($SS_{Within\ subject}$).

$SS_{Between\ subject}$ - Variation of individual subject's mean around grand mean and represents variation from individual to individual.

$SS_{Within\ subject}$ - Variation of individual's observation around respective mean. It is to note here that Between subject factor (SS_B) is included in $SS_{Between\ subject}$ whereas Within-subject factor (SS_W) and interaction between two factors ($SS_{Interaction}$) is in $SS_{Within\ subject}$.

Partitioning of Variances (Flow Chart 10)

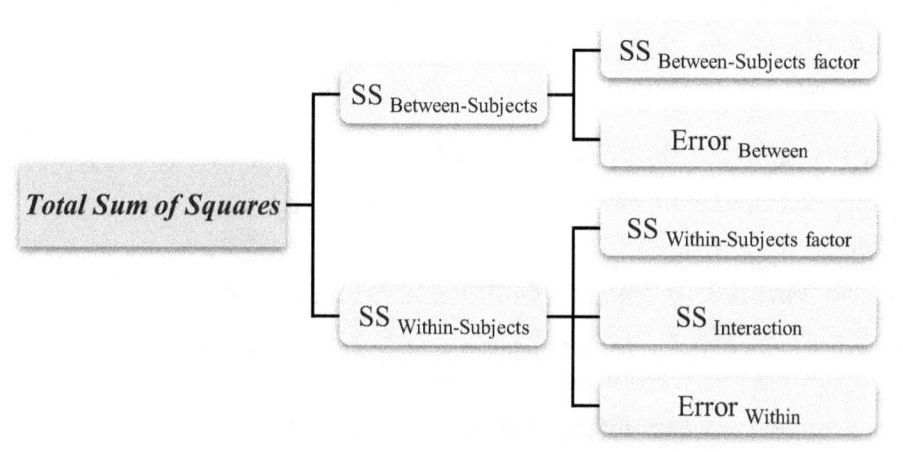

```
                              ┌── SS Between-Subjects factor
          ┌── SS Between-Subjects ──┤
          │                   └── Error Between
Total Sum │
of Squares│                   ┌── SS Within-Subjects factor
          └── SS Within-Subjects ───┼── SS Interaction
                              └── Error Within
```

Flow Chart 10: Variances in Mixed-Design ANOVA

Conducting Mixed ANOVA (Table 21-24)

Step 1: Calculate Grand mean and each individual mean (row wise)

Step 2: Calculate sum of square (SS)

$$SS_{total} = \Sigma(GM - individual\ value)^2$$
$$= \Sigma Number\ of\ observations\ of\ each\ subject$$
$$* (GM - each\ subject's\ mean)^2$$

$SS_{Within\ subject} = \Sigma(\text{Cell value row wise} - \text{Respective subject's mean})^2$

$SS_B = \Sigma$ *Number of observations in each subgroup*
$* (GM$
$- \text{Mean of subgroup of Between subject factor})^2$

$SS_{error(between)}$
$= \Sigma$ *Number of observations of each individual*
$* (\text{Each individual's mean}$
$- \text{Mean of subgroup of Between subject factor})^2$

Remember, $SS_{Between\ subject} = SS_B + SS_{error(between)}$

$SSw = \Sigma Number\ of\ participant * (GM - column\ mean)^2$ (Here, calculation column wise)

$SS_{Interaction} =$
Total variation due to all treatment groups $- SS_B - SS_W$
Total variation due to all treatment group
$= Subjects/group * (GM - Group\ mean)^2$

$SS_{error(within)} = SS_{Within\ subject} - SSw - SS_{interaction}$

Step 3: Calculate degree of freedom(df)

$df_{total} =$ *Total number of observations* $- 1$ $df_{Between\ subjects} =$ *Number of subjects* $- 1$

$df_B =$ *Number of levels of between subject factor* $- 1$

$df_{error(between)} = df_{Between\ subjects} - df_B$

$df_{Within\ subject} =$ *Total number of observations*
$-$ *Number of subjects*

$df_W =$ *Number of levels of within subject factor* $- 1$

$df_{interaction} = df_{BW} = df_B * df_W$

$df_{error(within)} = df_{Within\ subject} - df_W - df_{BW}$

Step 4: Calculate Mean sum square (MS)

MS for is obtained dividing SS by df. Calculation of MS for within subject factor, MS Interaction term and MS error (within) are same.

$MS_{Between\ subject\ factor} = \dfrac{SS_B}{df_B}$

$MS_{Within\ subject\ factor} = \dfrac{SS_W}{df_W}$ $MS_{interaction} = \dfrac{SS_{Interaction}}{df_{BW}}$

$MS_{error(between)} = \dfrac{SS_{error(between)}}{df_{error(between)}}$

$$MS_{error(Within)} = \frac{SS_{error(within)}}{df_{error\ (within)}}$$

Step 5: Calculate F value

$$F_{Between\ subject\ factor} = \frac{MS_{Between\ subject\ factor}}{MS_{error(between)}}$$

$$F_{Within\ subject\ factor} = \frac{MS_{Within\ subject\ factor}}{MS_{error(within)}}$$

$$F_{interaction} = \frac{MS_{interaction}}{MS_{error(within)}}$$

Interpretation: Find table value with corresponding degree of freedom and compare it with calculated F.

Skills on Statistical Calculation

Table 21: CRP Conc. in Two Different Drug Groups over Time

	ID	T1	T2	T3	Mean of individual	Error between
Drug A	1	7.0	4	1	4.0	0.4
	2	8.0	1	2	3.7	0.9
	3	9.0	4	5	6.0	2.0
Drug B	4	5.0	10	7	7.3	0.1
	5	9.0	6	3	6.0	1.0
	6	6.0	8	9	7.7	0.4
Mean of col		7.3	5.5	4.5		14.2
Mean Drug A	4.6					
Mean Drug B	7.0					
Grand Mean	5.8					

From the above table, we can also calculate the followings:
$SS_T = 137.1$, $SS_{Between\ subject} = 41.1$, $SS_B = 26.9$
$SS_{error\ (between)} = 14.2$, $SS_{Within\ subject} = 96.0$, $SS_W = 24.8$
$SS_{Interaction} = 32.3$, $SS_{Error\ (within)} = 38.9$.

Treatment groups with their respective mean in Table 23 below.

Table 22: Mixed ANOVA (Partitioning of Variances)

	SST	SS Between subject	SS Within subject
SS	137.11	41.11	96.00
DF	18-1=17	6-1=5	18-6=12

Table 23: Treatment groups in mixed ANOVA

AT1	AT2	AT3	BT1	BT2	BT3
7	4	1	5	10	7
8	1	2	9	6	3
9	4	5	6	8	9
8.00	3.00	3.50	6.67	8.00	6.33

$SS\ Interaction = Total\ variation - SS_B - SSw = 32.3$

$SS_{error(within)} = SS_{Within\ subject} - SSw - SS_{Interaction} = 38.9$

Table 24: Reporting Table of Mixed ANOVA

	SS	DF	MS	F
$SS_{Between\ subject}$				
SS_B	26.9	2-1=1	26.89/1 = 26.9	7.5
$SS_{error(between)}$	14.2	5-1=4	14.2/4=3.7	
$SS_{Within\ subject}$				
SS_W	24.8	3-1=2	24.78/2 = 12.4	2.5
$SS_{interaction}$	32.3	1*2=2	32.33/2=16.2	3.3
$SS_{error(within)}$	38.9	12-2-2=8	38.89/8 = 4.9	

Interpretation (Table 24)

F value of Effect of Drugs with df (1,4) from table is 7.71 (α=0.05) is < Calculated value 7.5. So, Effect of Drugs significant. [From excel, F.INV.RT (0.05,1,4) returns 7.71]. F value of Time with df (2,8) from table is 4.46 (α=0.05) is > Calculated value 2.5. So, Effect of Time period has no significant effect. [From excel, F.INV.RT (0.05,2,8) returns 4.458]. F value of Drug* Time (Interaction) with df (2,8) from table is 4.46 (α=0.05) is > Calculated value 3.3. So, no interaction effect. In excel, run two factor ANOVA without replication (for repeated measure ANOVA) and two factor ANOVA with replication for analysis of between group design. Reporting table construction requires some modification as well as composing two tables.

Example 1: Researcher enrolled 60 newborn babies with jaundice and randomly assigned to two treatment group. Group I received Phototherapy and Group II received Phenobarbitone. Duration of study 72hrs. He is eager to know whether bilirubin concentration varies in two groups over different time period? Bilirubin estimated Day 0, Day 2 and Day 3.

Section 4.7: Within-Within ANOVA

Understanding Withing-Within ANOVA

A within-within-subject ANOVA is used when a dependent variable is measured over time when participants have been subjected to two or more treatment. Here, we measure any two within-subject factors in subjects and try to understand whether there is an interaction between these factors.

Researcher selected five participants and tried to understand whether change in cholesterol concentration is different over time (say in three time points) with two cholesterol lowering drugs (new and standard). This can be stated in another way like this: Does the changes in cholesterol concentration at the different time points depends on drug they were prescribed? Thus, interaction effect can be analyzed. Here, there are two within subject factors (time, drug) and dependent variable is serum cholesterol conc. This type of ANOVA is also known as two factor repeated measure ANOVA.

Assumptions
- ❖ Normal distribution of data in each group and No Outlier
- ❖ Variances of the differences between two groups (two time periods) are equal- Assumption of Sphericity

Partitioning of Variances (Flow Chart 11)

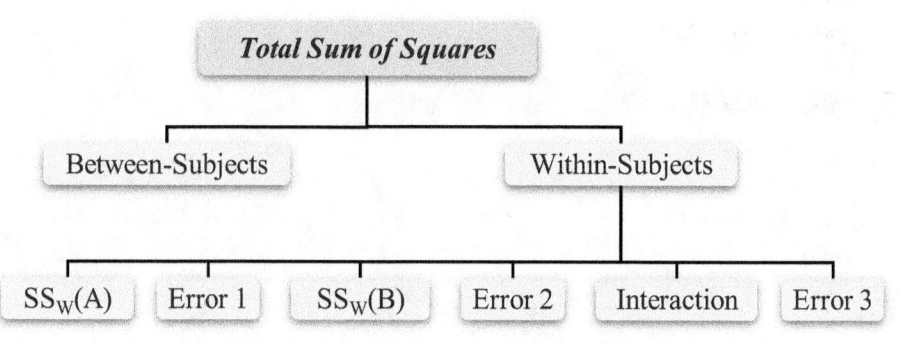

```
                    Total Sum of Squares
                    /                \
           Between-Subjects      Within-Subjects
                |              /     |      \
          SS_W(A)  Error 1  SS_W(B)  Error 2  Interaction  Error 3
```

Flow Chart 11: Partitioning of Variances

Biostatistics in Health Research

Steps of Data Collection

Step 1: Five subjects recruited
Step 2: Standard drug given
Step 3: Cholesterol conc. measured in Time 1, Time 2, Time 3
Step 4: Wash out period and same subjects received new drug
Step 5: Cholesterol conc. measured in Time 1, Time 2, Time 3

Data Presentation (Table 25): Cholesterol conc. over time periods

Table 25: Two-Way ANOVA Repeated Measures on Both Factors

Subject	Standard drug				New drug		
	T_1	T_2	T_3	Wash out period	T_1	T_2	T_3
Sub 1							
Sub 2							
Sub 3							
Sub 4							
Sub 5							

Analysis (Overview)
- Mean value of cholesterol conc. at different time periods
- Checking for outlier and testing normality
- Profile plot for interaction between Time and treatment
- Descriptive statistics (mean, SD, standard error)

Table 26: Reporting Within-Within ANOVA

Sources of Variation	SS	df	MS	F cal	F Table
Between subjects					
Within-subjects					
Within-subject factor A					
Error 1					
Within-subject factor B					
Error 2					
Interaction					
Error 3					
Total					

Section 4.8: FAQ on ANOVA

1. Why doing ANOVA instead of doing multiple t tests?
2. Define independent and dependent variable.
   Independent variable-Variable that is manipulated by researchers and has an effect on dependent variable. Dependent variable is measured and tested.
3. Which term captures variances in different ANOVA?
   Sum of Squares
4. How the following terms are different from each other:
   Homogeneity of variances, Homoscedasticity and Sphericity
5. What do you mean by (OFAT)?
   Here we test factors, or causes, one at a time instead of multiple factors simultaneously. Disadvantages:
   - Inefficient and time consuming
   - Huge experimental runs
   - Interaction effect cannot be studied
6. How variances are partitioned in different types of ANOVA?
7. What do you mean by Sphericity?
8. What is residual? What are the different types of residuals? How they differ from each other? How to calculate each of them. State their applications.
9. Name different types of Study design that detects interaction effects. What are the different Statistical tests to detect interaction effects in different types of study design? (Prepare Table)

MANOVA (Multivariate Analysis of Variance)

It is an extension of ANOVA that includes two or more DV instead of one DV. Here DV are combined to form a 'new' DV and test the differences between the groups of the IV. So far, we have discussed, DV is continuous and IV is qualitative in nature. Here, there may be one or more IV which is categorized into groups and two or more DV which are continuous variables. In one-way MANOVA, there is one IV and one or more DV. When there are two IV, it is known as two-way MANOVA. MANCOVA includes covariates.

Here, the researcher wants to know whether the composite form (mean vector) of the DV varies across levels of IV. We calculate test statistic such as Wilk's lambda, Pillai's trace, Hotelling's trace and Roy's Largest root. If found significant, we go for follow up test such as one way ANOVA, Discriminant function analysis to see which DV is responsible for such significance. Its assumptions involve very complex process and requires help of software. In fact, whole procedure (assumption testing and analysis) is carried out with the software. Beginners should learn the situations where MANOVA should be conducted and should take the help of a statistician.

Example 1: In a study, 60 persons were randomized into three groups (20 participants in each group) and received three different diet charts (Diet plan A, Diet plan B, Diet plan C). With these plan, Body weight loss, Serum Cholesterol recorded for each participant. Investigator wants to study whether the Body weight reduction and serum cholesterol differs among different diet plan.

Example 2: Three Stress Reducing Techniques are being applied on 120 participants. There are three groups (40 participants in each group). Each group is subject to one particular technique. Study duration is 3 months. At the end, researcher collected information on Anxiety score and Systolic blood pressure. Study aimed to investigate whether Anxiety score and Systolic blood pressure differs among groups receiving Stress reducing techniques.

MANOVA Table

Subject ID	Diet Plan	Weight Loss	Cholesterol
1	Plan A		
2			
3			
4			
5			
6	Plan B		
7			
8			
9			
10			

Section 5: Chi-Square Test

Introduction

Sometimes studies are carried out to find if there is an association between two qualitative variables. Responses like Yes / No, failure / success Response / No-response, cured / not cured falls in this category. Null hypothesis states two variables are not related whereas alternate hypothesis states variable is interdependent.

Chi-square is calculated from values for each cell response (observed and expected value) and is given by

$x^2 = \sum \frac{(O-E)^2}{E}$, here $df =$ (Column - 1) × (Row- 1). If calculated value is greater than table value, we reject null hypothesis. When binary data are used, we should go for Yate's correction to have accurate results. After correction formula becomes $x^2 = \sum \frac{\{|O-E|-0.5\}^2}{E}$. Here 0.5 is subtracted from absolute diff. between observed value and expected value. After deduction of 0.5, if the value comes negative, we take it as zero. Phi and Cramer's V are measures of the strength of association between two categorical variables but a more common and possibly more useful measure of effect size for categorical data is OR.

Assumptions
- Variables under study is nominal
- Expected frequency for each category of the variable is at least 5. Although it is acceptable in larger contingency tables to have up to 20% of expected frequencies below 5, the result is a loss of statistical power (test may fail to detect a genuine effect). In larger contingency tables no expected frequencies should be below 1 and consider Fisher's test in this situation.
- Independence of observations

Applications
- Test to find statistically significant difference in two or more proportions.
- To test association between two variables (whether two variables are related or independent).

Biostatistics in Health Research

- Test for goodness of fit- Comparing observed frequencies with expected or theoretical frequencies.

Types of Chi-square Test
- Chi-Square Test of Independence
- Chi-Square Test of Goodness of -Fit- Whether observed distribution is similar to known distribution.
- Chi-Square Test for Trend- There are two variables. One variable is binary and other variable is categorized into three or more and ordered in nature.
- Chi-Square Test of Proportion
- Likelihood Chi-Square Test
- Mc Nemar Test

Chi-square Statistic in Goodness of Fit

Problem 1: A company claims that their new product Drug A has 90% cure rate. But on trial with that drug on 90 patients showed 70% cure rate (Table 27). Do you agree with the company what they claim?

Table 27: Chi- square (Goodness of Fit)

	Cured	Not cured	Total
Observed	63	27	90
Expected	81	9	90
Total	144	36	180

$\chi^2 = (63-81)^2/81 + (27-9)^2/9 = 4+36 = 40$ (Table 26). Here df is 1, table value at 1 df 3.84 at 5% level of significance. You can get table value of test statistics in excel function CHI.INV.RT(0.05,1). As calculated value is > table value, we can't agree with the claim.

Here $\chi^2 = \sum \dfrac{(\text{Observed frequency - Expected frequency})^2}{\text{Expected frequency}}$

Degree of freedom = (Column − 1) × (Row−1). There are two columns and two rows. So, df becomes one.

Problem 2: 45 patients of chronic backache are divided into three groups and received three different analgesics. Mean time of pain relief reported from three groups: 20 min, 30 min, 40 min. Can you conclude that difference is due to medication or due to chance?

Chi-square Test of Independence

Problem: In Table 28 below, trial results given for a drug compared with a placebo. Test whether outcome is independent of treatment.

Table 28: Trial Results

Treatment	Outcome Died	Outcome Survived	Total
Drug	5	75	80
Placebo	10	40	50
Total	15	115	130

Table 29: Expected Frequencies

Treatment	Outcome Died	Outcome Survived	Total
Drug	9.24	70.76	80
Placebo	5.76	44.24	50
Total	15	115	130

Step 1: State null hypothesis that there is no difference in outcome in two groups

Step 2: Prepare contingency table

Step 3: Calculate expected frequency for each cell (Table 29)

$$\text{Expected frequency} = \frac{(\text{Row total} \times \text{Column total})}{\text{Grand total}}$$

Step 4: Compute χ^2

Step 5: Find out degree of freedom

Step 6: Find table value of chi-square with particular df = 3.84

Step 7: Compare table value with calculated value

Step 8: Draw conclusion.

If calculated value is greater than table value, we reject null hypothesis and conclude that they differ.

$\chi^2 = 1.938 + 0.254 + 3.121 + 0.405 = 5.718$

Here df is 1, table value comes to 3.84 which is less than calculated value. So, we conclude that there is significant difference. (In excel, CHISQ.INV.RT(p value, df) returns 3.84)

Yate's Correction

Now as the Chi-square distribution is continuous whereas 2*2 table is discrete (binomial) in nature, there may be error doing χ^2 test.

To avoid such error, Yate's correction is done where 0.5 is subtracted from the absolute difference between observed and expected frequency, then squared and divided by expected frequency. Finally, added to get Chi-square value for each cell. Controversies exist among statisticians regarding its usefulness, we suggest that beginners should be familiar with this procedure.

Procedure

Step 1: State null and alternate hypothesis
Step 2: Prepare contingency table
Step 3: Calculate expected frequency for each cell
Step 4: Compute χ^2
Step 5: Find out degree of freedom
Step 6: Find table value of chi-square with particular df = 3.84
Step 7: Compare table value with calculated value
Step 8: Draw conclusion.

Interpretation: If calculated value is > table value, we reject null hypothesis and conclude that they differ.

$\chi^2 = 1.507 + 0.1966 + 2.412 + 0.3146 = 4.432$. Here df is 1, table value comes to 3.84 which is less than calculated value. So, we conclude that there is significant difference.

Chi-square Test of Proportions

Problem: In a drug trial, Drug A has 90% and Drug B has 70% cure rate. In first group 1, there were 150 subjects and in group 2, there were 80 patients (Table 30). Are they treatment equally effective?

Step 1: State null hypothesis and alternate hypothesis
Step 2: Prepare contingency table
Step 3: Calculate expected frequency for each cell (Table 31)
Step 4: Compute χ^2
Step 5: Find out df
Step 6: Find table value of chi-square with particular df

Step 7: Compare table value with calculated value

Step 8: Draw conclusion. If calculated value is greater than table value, we reject null hypothesis and conclude that they differ.

Table 30: Treatment & Outcome

Treatment	Disease status		Total
	Cured	Not cured	
Drug A	135	15	150
Drug B	56	24	80
Total	191	39	230

Table 31: Expected Frequency

Treatment	Disease status		Total
	Cured	Not cured	
Drug A	111.52	38.48	150
Drug B	59.48	20.52	80
Total	171	59	230

$\chi^2 = 0.874117915 + 4.280936 + 1.63897109 + 8.026756 = 14.82078$

Table value with df 1 is 3.84. As calculated value is less than table value, we conclude that they do not differ at 0.05.

Log Linear Regression

It is used when there are three or more categorical variables and we select model which is best fit for the data. Interaction between variables can be tested in this procedure. We usually perform with the help of a statistical software. Association between two categorical variables can also be tested and yields same information.

Mc Nemar Test

Observations are recorded on dichotomous scale using same participants on two occasions. Thus, its applications are very similar to paired sample t test, only difference being data are binary.

Applications of McNemar Test
- ❖ Difference between two different conditions
- ❖ Changes over two time periods
- ❖ Differences in matched pairs

Suppose, an awareness program about health hazards was conducted among 100 adult participants. Some were smokers and some non-smokers. After the program, we again counted number of smokers and non-smokers, in addition to that we counted who changed their habit (i.e., smoker to non-smoker, non-smoker to smoker). Our interest is whether the awareness program has significant impact on habit.

Null and Alternate Hypothesis

H_0: Awareness program has no impact on smoking habit
H_1: Awareness program has significant impact on smoking habit

Taking another example where opinions were recorded among 150 faculties in favor and against Competency based medical education (CBME). After that an awareness program was conducted among those faculties. Responses in the form of favor, against as well as change in opinion were recorded (Table 32a).

Table 32a: Introducing CBME in Medical Colleges

Before Sensitization	After Sensitization	
	Against CBME	In Favor of CBME
Against CBME	A	B
In Favor of CBME	C	D

Statistical Procedure: In descriptive section, we report proportion of faculties for a particular characteristic. In addition, faculties change their opinion (C = in favor to against, B = Against to in favor.). Here, test statistic χ^2 after continuity correction is given by $\chi^2 = \frac{(|B-C|-1)^2}{B+C}$ with one degree of freedom. If the calculated value > table value (Critical value), null hypothesis is rejected and alternate hypothesis is accepted. B, C represent disagreement or discordant pairs. If the total of B, C is < 20, then we report exact significance assuming binomial distribution. When Chi-square distribution is followed (i.e., B, C total > 20), we report asymptotic significance. In binomial distribution (B, C total < 20), assuming 0.5 probability and smaller between B & C is to be used, total trials equal B+C with excel function BINORM.DIST. Multiply with 2 to have two tailed result.

Cochran Q Test

This type of test is applicable when three or more groups are used but subjects are same in all groups (matched samples, repeated measures) and recorded response is binary in nature. It is an extension of Mc Nemar test.

Null Hypothesis: Proportion of scores across all groups are same
Alternate Hypothesis: Score of at least one treatment group differs
Suppose three drugs are being given in 6 subjects after wash out period, response recorded Cured/Not Cured (Table 32b).

Table 32b: Cochran Q Table Format

Participant ID	Drug A	Drug B	Drug C	Total
Participant 1				
Participant 2				
Participant 3				
Participant 4				
Participant 5				
Participant 6				
Total				

Procedure

Step 1: Calculate each subject's total score
Step 2: Square each subject's total score (P1, P2, P3….)
Step 3: Add (say P^2)
Step 4: Add scores in each treatment group (T1, T2, T3….)
Step 5: Add total and square it say T^2
Step 6: Now calculate Q (Formula given below)
Step 7: Calculate df (Number of groups-1), say number of groups k
Step 8: Find Table value of test statistic using Chi square distribution with particular df and p value. Use =CHISQ.INV.RT(p value, df).
Step 9: Compare calculated value with the table of test statistics.
Step 10: Reject Null hypothesis if Q> table value.

$$Q = \frac{(k-1)[k \times P^2 - T^2]}{k \times T - T^2}$$

Section 6: Non-parametric Test

Understanding Non-parametric Test

Parameter is a measurement of population. In a parametric test, we test hypotheses about a population parameter. Before performing parametric test, we must test for the assumptions. These assumptions are normal distribution of population, homogeneity of variances, there should be no outlier. Observations are independent.

If these assumptions are not met, we carry out non parametric test. Here we assume that population from where data are collected need not be normally distributed. We do not test hypotheses about population parameter, and it is not necessarily be random samples from normally distributed population (Table 33). Data in non-parametric test are qualitative or categorical whereas in parametric test, they are quantitative in nature. Large samples are difficult to be analyzed with non-parametric test and also multiple factor analysis along with interaction effects cannot be tested with this procedure.

Table 33: Difference Between Parametric and Non-parametric Test

Parametric test	Nonparametric test
Normal distribution of population	No assumption about population
Homogeneity of variance /absence of	Not required
Large samples can be tested	Difficult to test
Quantitative data	Qualitative data
More Powerful	Less powerful
Tests Multiple factors and interaction effects	No comparable statistical technique exists
Examples: Student t test, ANOVA	Mann Whitney test, χ^2 test

If any sample is amenable to both types of tests, we carry out parametric test as it is more powerful. Different non parametric equivalent tests are here presented in the Table 34.

Table 34: Non-parametric Tests and Parametric Alternatives

Nonparametric test	Parametric alternative
Sign test	One sample t-test
Friedman test	Repeated measure ANOVA
Kruskal-Wallis's test	One-way ANOVA
Mann-Whitney test	Independent samples t-test
Wilcoxon signed rank test	Paired samples t-test
Spearman Rank Correlation	Correlation Coefficient

Skills on Statistical Calculation

Wilcoxon Signed Rank Test in Excel (Table 35)

Table 35: Excel Table for Wilcoxon Signed Rank Test

Before	After	Sign Diff	ABS Diff	Rank Diff	Sign Ranks	Sum(+) Ranks	Sum(-)Ranks	ABS Smaller Sum

Step 1: Column 1 and Column 2 shows paired data

Step 2: Create a column (Column3) next to data named Sign of difference. Type =Sign ( ) and select respective rows for difference.

Step 3: Column 4 calculates absolute difference

Step 4: Column 5 shows ranking that deals with ties (observations with same score) also by typing Rank.avg (place $ sign in reference range)

Step 4: Column 6 shows sign of ranks by multiplying with Col 3 & 5

Step 5: Calculate sum of (+), (-) ranks typing Sumif (range, criteria, [sum_range]) and place ($) in range and sum_range.

Step 6: Consider absolute value for both and take smaller value as test statistic

Step 7: Whether the smaller value is really smaller or not, we are to find critical value from table with appropriate sample size. If test statistic is lower than table value, reject null hypothesis.

Mann Whitney Test (Table 36)

Step 1: Column 1 and Column 2 shows unpaired data

Step 2: Create two columns (Col 3&4) next to observed data named RANK 1 and RANK 2. Ranking deals with ties (observations with same score) by typing Rank.avg in excel (place $ in reference range)

Step 3: Column 5&6 shows sum of RANK1 and RANK2

Step 4: Go to the table where left side shows smaller sample and upper side shows larger values and determine whether smaller rank sum is < the table value or not. If small, then reject null hypothesis.

Table 36: Analysis Table of Mann Whitney Test

Gr 1	Gr 2	RANK 1	RANK 2	Sum RANK1	Sum RANK2

Spearman Rank Correlation Coefficient

Step 1: Column 1 and Column 2 shows data of two variables

Step 2: We will create two columns (Column 3&4) next to observed data named RANK 1 and RANK 2. Ranking deals with ties (observations with same score) by typing Rank.avg in excel (place dollar sign in reference range)

Step 3: Use function CORREL () using RANK1 and RANK2

Step 4: Go to table to determine whether correlation coefficient function is significant or not.

Chapter 7: Study Design

Section 1: Common Types of Study Design

Cross Over Design

This is a very popular design in clinical trial. Each subject receives all types of treatments. The orders in which they receive treatment are randomized. After receiving one treatment in period 1, there is wash out period and then receives another treatment in period 2. The order of treatment administration is called a sequence and the time of a treatment is called a period. Usually, two treatments are studied (Image 1). In parallel design, patients are randomized to a treatment and remain on that treatment throughout the trial (Table 1). Inter individual variability is reduced as each subject serves as their own control. Effect of confounding is reduced. Only chronic and stable diseases are studied. Treatment should not cure but alleviate the disease. Wash out period should be sufficient (five half-lives of the drug) to avoid carry over effect. It exists when the effect of the treatment from the previous time period on the response affects the current time period. Thus, it may introduce bias in the study. This effect is seen in different teaching methods and different types of psychotherapy. It is a type of cross over design for r-period, r-treatment and is unique as each treatment occurs only once within each sequence and once within each period.

Applications
- ❖ Chronic diseases (asthma, arthritis) which are stable
- ❖ Mainly used for Bio equivalence study, phase 1. Not preferred in Acute disease and Vaccine trial.

Advantages of Cross Over Design
- Study participants serve as their own control
- Variability reduced, so precision increased
- Small sample size
- Influence of the confounder decreased
- Subjects have opportunity to receive all types of treatments

Disadvantages of Cross Over Design
- ❖ Unwilling subjects are not allowed in the study

- Diseases which are stable and chronic are studied
- Subjected to carry over effect and period effect
- Takes more time to complete
- Problem if drug resistance, drop out, hit and run drug etc.

Table 1: Comparison between Parallel and Crossover Design

Parallel Design	Cross Over Design
Each group receives different	Same treatment
Large sample size	Small sample size
Acute diseases are preferred	Chronic & stable
No carry over effect	Carry over effect present
Takes less time	Takes long time
Inter individual variation present	Absent
Effect of confounding present	Absent

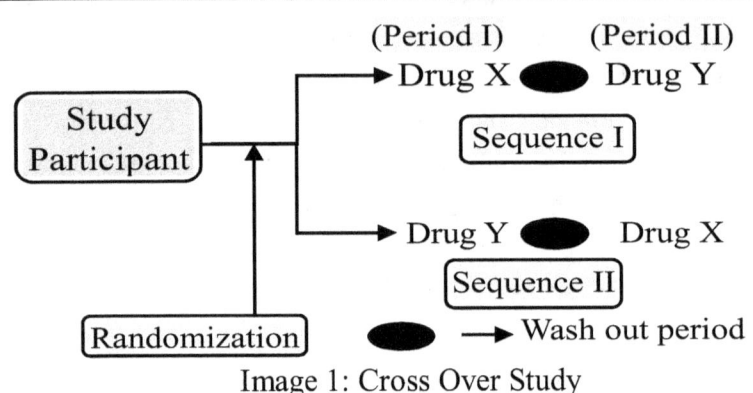

Image 1: Cross Over Study

Analysis

Number of Treatments: Any number of treatments can be analyzed but here we are going with 2 or 3 treatments for the beginners.

Sequence: If you have 2 treatments (X, Y) then number of sequences 2 (XY, YX), if three treatments (X, Y, Z) then number of sequences 6 (XYZ, YZX, ZXY, YXZ, XZY, ZYX). Number of sequences equals K! (Factorial K). So, with four treatments 4*3*2*1 =24

Period: Equals number of treatments

Nature of Data: Continuous, Binary or Ordinal

Effects that can be studied:

Main effect- Effect of treatment on outcome

Carry over effect-Does the effect of a treatment in one period persists in next period?

Sequence effect- Does the order of treatment has impact on outcome?
Period effect- Does the outcome differs across periods and not related to treatment?
Interaction effect- Two interactions can be studied if anyone is Treatment by Period (Tests whether effect of treatments depends on which period the treatment is administered) and another is Sequence by Period (Whether order of treatment has different effect depending upon the period).

Assumptions to be fulfilled:
- ❖ Homogeneity of variances
- ❖ Normally distributed data

From the above discussion, it is obvious that for analysis purpose we have to consider first assumption. Then consider number of treatments and nature of data (Continuous, Binary or Ordinal).Type of statistical tests differ if assumptions are not met. In situations where more than two treatments are administered, complex procedure may be required. Analysis through software such as SPSS will be helpful. Beginners will also be able to analyze two or more than two treatment groups using simple parametric tests, non-parametric test and regression analysis. In all cases, all the Five effects are to be tested and interpreted carefully

Analysis
- ❖ Parametric tests: Independent t test, paired t test, ANOVA, Repeated measure ANOVA, Two Way ANOVA
- ❖ Non parametric tests.
- ❖ Regression procedure: Linear, Binary logistic and Ordinal logistic regression and Linear Mixed Effect model. Friends, don't worry, proceed step by step and enjoy.

Latin Square Design (LSD)

It is a type of cross over design where there are three or more treatments. There are equal number of rows and columns and each treatment occurs only once in row and column. Here
Number of Treatments=Number of Rows= Number of Columns
Normally LSD is a three-factor experiment where it is assumed that there is no interaction between rows, columns and treatments which means

that they affect dependent variable independently. As the interaction term is ignored, number of experiments is reduced. Thus, we can say that LSD is a main effect only design. In practice, influence of interactions is merged within the error term in ANOVA table. As a result, value of F is reduced because error is in denominator in F calculation and the chance of getting significant result is lessened (Table 2). Row and column are two sources of variations that we can control in LSD.

Advantages of Latin Square Design
- ✓ Simple procedure
- ✓ No of experiments reduced compared to factorial design
- ✓ Control two sources of variation

Steps of Analysis (Table 3)
Here we are seeing the effect of a particular treatment and suppose it has three levels. Now there are two other factors we can control in this analysis, say factor A and factor B but we are assuming there are no interactions between factor A, factor B and treatment. Placing factor A in row, factor B in column, we can present the design as given below assuming there are three levels for both factors. As per criteria of LS design, each treatment occurs only once in row and column. T_1, T_2, T_3 are levels of treatment.

Table 2: Latin Square Design

	Factor B		
Factor A	T_1	T_2	T_3
	T_2	T_3	T_1
	T_3	T_1	T_2

Table 3 of analysis is like three-way ANOVA. We have seen how to prepare ANOVA table for two factors. It looks similar to that one. SS for treatment factor, factor A, factor B will have to calculated along with df. MSS is obtained dividing SS by df and F value by dividing MSS by Error MSS. If calculated F is > table value, we reject null hypothesis and accept alternate hypothesis.

Table 3: ANOVA Table of Latin Square Design

	SS	df	MSS	F
Factor A		3-1		MSS factor A / MSS error
Factor B		3-1		MSS factor B / MSS error
Treatment		3-1		MSS treatment / MSS error
Error		8-(2+2+2)		
Total		3^2 -1		

Factorial Design

Factorial design is a type of research design that helps to investigate the main and interaction effects between two or more factors (independent variables) and on one or more outcome variable(s). Factors may be quantitative or qualitative. The main effect of a factor is defined as change in response produced in different level of a factor. If the difference in response between the levels of one factor is not same at all levels of the other factor, there is an interaction between the factors. Graphs are useful in interpreting interactions, though it must be proved statistically. Parallel lines in a plot signify no interaction. Main effects have little practical meaning in presence of interaction. A significant interaction often masks the significance of main effects.

Advantages

They are more efficient than one-factor-at-a-time (OFAT) experiments. Factorial designs allow the effects of a factor at several levels of the other factors, yielding conclusions that are valid over a range of experimental conditions. A factorial design is necessary when interactions are suspected to avoid misleading conclusions. Factorial designs are more efficient than compared to OFAT experiments and provide more information at similar or lower cost. They can find optimal conditions faster than OFAT.

Full Factorial Design

2^3 – Here no of factors 3, each has 2 levels. No of experiments 8
3^2 -here no of factors 2, each has 3 levels. No of experiments 9
Disadvantages: If the number of factors is large, number of experiments increase and leads to an unmanageable situation. In that case, we use fractional factorial design.

Biostatistics in Health Research

Fractional Factorial Design
Large number of factors is studied with lesser number of experiments efficiently. 2^{4-1} design means with total of 8 experimental runs, 4 factors can be studied. Higher than 2nd order interactions are not taken into account as these interactions are very rarely significant. This type of design is considered when number of factors 5 or more. Studying effect on blood pressure with 2 doses of losartan on both sexes is a simple example of factorial design where dependent variable is blood pressure (quantitative). Gender and Drug are two factors where gender has 2 levels and Drug losartan has 2 dose levels. Design will be 2^2, total number of experiments being 4. Analysis by ANOVA or regression.

Carry Over Effect
Carry Over Effect is showing the effect of one previous experimental condition which is affecting current experiment. Suppose, a person is given a numerical chart to remember to test his memory with a placebo and result is noted. Again, after few days same patient with test drug is given the same chart. Now due to carry over effect of previous experiment with same chart, he may falsely show high memory. Let us take another example. A group of participants are being treated with Drug A and then same subjects are being treated with Drug B, now when we measure the effect of Drug B, we get influence of Drug A on Drug B outcome. Carry over effect is common in cross over design. Sufficient wash out period is essential to overcome this effect. In case of drug, it is important to consider half-life. Linear mixed model, ANOVA and Paired t test may help to overcome this type of effect.

Sequence Effect
Sequence effect refers to influence of order of treatments on outcome. Suppose participants receive Drug A first and then Drug B (sequence AB), effect of Drug B differs if given first then Drug A (sequence BA). This is due to difference in treatment order. Randomization of treatment order and using appropriate study design may nullify such effect.

Section 2: FAQ on Study Design

1. Write difference between Type of study and Study design?
2. Discuss different types of One Factor Experimental Design.
3. How Repeated measures and Cross over design differs?

   Both conditions are aimed to study effects of multiple conditions/treatments using same subjects. Repeated measure design may not necessarily study effect of treatments, simply observe effects of different conditions over time. There is no wash out period. Subjects serves as their own control, thus controlling within-subject variability. Repeated measure design is commonly used in educational research and psychology. Studying effect of Drug A on CRP conc. in a group of participants in first, second and six weeks after therapy is an example of repeated measure design. Multiple treatments are administered in a cross over design with wash out period in between treatments. Sequence effect and carry over effect is there (Be careful). Controls between-subject variability.

4. What is Standard and Definitive Screening Design?
5. What is Spillover Effect?

   Intervention in one group of people may affect other groups not receiving intervention. Introduction of new teaching learning strategy as per Medical Education Technology in one medical college may affect behaviour of faculties and students in other medical colleges. Thus, concept of spillover effect is essential to know to have true interpretation of an intervention.

Chapter 8: Correlation and Regression

Section 1: Correlation

Concept behind Correlation

It measures the magnitude and direction of association between two variables. Scatter diagram is used to describe the relationship between the two variables. If pattern of points on the graph shows the linear trend or path, we say there is a linear relationship. This plot is essential when we go for prediction or regression analysis. Correlation coefficient(r) quantitatively expresses the magnitude and direction of association. Underlying concept of r is the ratio of variability of the variables combined and separately.

$$r = \frac{\text{Degree to which both variables vary simultaneously}}{\text{Degree to which both variables vary separately}} = \frac{\text{Covariance (X,Y)}}{\text{Variability of both variables vary separately}}$$

Properties of Correlation
- ❖ r lies between -1 and +1. $r = 0$ -no relationship.
- ❖ Sign indicates direction of relationship.
- ❖ No units of measurements
- ❖ Interpretation of r is within the range of values of variables in the sample- results cannot be generalized.
- ❖ Cause and effect relationship can't be established.

Assumption of Correlation
- ❖ Both variables are quantitative
- ❖ Linear relationship and no outlier
- ❖ Normal distribution of at least one of the variables
- ❖ No paired observation (Independence of observation)

Applications: Regression analysis/Validity of a test/Reliability of a test
Types of Correlation: It is of two types: Linear and Non-linear. Linear correlation may be positive (both variables move in same direction), negative (variables move in opposite direction) and zero correlation.

Positive correlation

Negative correlation

Curvilinear relationship

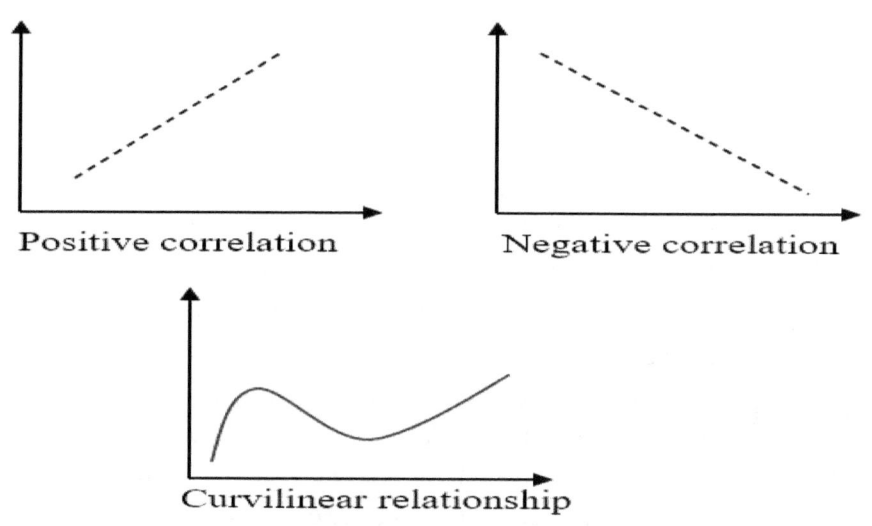

Image 1: Different Types of Relationship

Skill on Statistical Calculation

Suppose there are two variables X and Y (Continuous), then

$$r = \frac{Co\ variance\ (X,Y)}{(SDx * SDy)}$$ where $Covar\ (X, Y) = \frac{\Sigma(X-\bar{X})(Y-\bar{Y})}{n-1}$

$$SDx = \sqrt{\frac{\Sigma(X-\bar{X})^2}{(n-1)}}, SDy = \sqrt{\frac{\Sigma(Y-\bar{Y})^2}{(n-1)}}$$

($\bar{X}, \bar{Y}$ are the mean and SDx and SDy represent SD of X and Y).

Different information required to calculate r is shown in Table 1 where excel will help us very much.

Procedure

Table 1: Correlation Table

X	Y	$X-\bar{X}$	$Y-\bar{Y}$	$(X-\bar{X})(Y-\bar{Y})$	$(X-\bar{X})^2$	$(Y-\bar{Y})^2$

Step 1: Calculate mean of the variables X and Y

Step 2: Find difference of each value from their respective mean $X-\bar{X}, Y-\bar{Y}$

Step 3: Calculate Co variance. Covariance calculation is available in Excel function form as COVARIANCE.P and COVARIANCE.S)

Step 4: SD of each variable

Step 5: $r = \frac{\sum(X-\bar{X})(Y-\bar{Y})}{\sqrt{\sum(X-\bar{X})^2} \times \sqrt{\sum(Y-\bar{Y})^2}}$

n-1 will be cancelled out from both numerator and denominator. Using Excel function, r = CORREL (). If the assumption of normality is not met or if one of the variables is ordinal in nature, then Spearman's rank correlation coefficient which is non parametric equivalent of r. Sometimes, relationship involves more than two variables such as partial and multiple correlation.

Partial Correlation

Measures strength of relationship between two variables after controlling the effect of other variables and thus removes confounding effect of other variables. If we want to find relationship between A & B after controlling for the effect of C, then relationship can be expressed mathematically as

$$r_{AB.C} = \frac{r_{AB} - r_{AC} \cdot r_{BC}}{\sqrt{(1 - r_{AC}^2)(1 - r_{BC}^2)}}$$

There are other methods of controlling effect of third variable such as Multiple Regression, ANCOVA, Stratification and Matching.

Non-parametric Correlation

Non-parametric type of correlation is used when assumptions of parametric correlation are not met. There are two non-parametric type of correlation: Spearman rank correlation and Kendall's Tau. Assumptions: Data is ordinal or continuous (that can be ranked), each pair of observations are independent (not correlated with other pairs) and variables are in monotonic relationship (when one increases, other also increases or decreases consistently but not constant increase or decrease). Spearman correlation is applicable for small to moderate sample size but preferred in large samples, sensitive to outlier, it can handle ties (identical values in data). Kendall's tau is preferred in small samples and when there are many tied ranks. Method of calculation of correlation is different in two types. Kendall's tau is more suitable thanspearman rank correlation in cases of outlier.

Section 2: Regression Analysis

Section 2.1: Linear Regression

Concept of Regression

In some situation, with the help of sample values, we predict the value of DV in the form of an equation. In case of regression, we can predict the value of DV with the help of one or more IV in the form of an equation which in its simplest form is represented by $y = a + bx$. In case of multiple IV, $y = a + b_1x_1 + b_2x_2 + b_3x_3 + b_nx_n$ (y is DV and x is IV).

a = Y intercept of regression line of Y on X
b = Regression coefficient of Y on X (slope/gradient of the line).

In case of correlation, there is no such concept of DV. Here in regression, to obtain straight line, we apply principle of least square which states that sum of squares of differences between observed and corresponding estimated value here is minimum. Regression coefficient is nothing but the change in DV y for unit change in IV x which is obtained mathematically.

$$b = \frac{\text{Covariance}(x,y)}{\text{Variance}(x)} = \frac{\sum(X-\bar{X})(Y-\bar{Y})}{\sum(X-\bar{X})^2}$$

$a = \bar{y} - b\bar{x}$ (Value of y when $x = 0$). Here (n-1) is being cancelled out from both numerator and denominator. Using excel function, type Slope and type Intercept to get b and a easily. Table 2 shows how to calculate data in a stepwise manner for regression analysis.

Table 2: Regression Analysis Table

X	Y	Y_{model} $= a + bx$	$SS_{residual}$ $= (Y - Y_{model})^2$	$SS_{regression}$ $= (\bar{Y} - Y_{model})^2$

Skill Development (Table 2,3 and Image 2)

Mathematical equation: Calculate slope(b), intercept (a) and frame mathematical equation as $y = a + bx$. Also calculate Predicted value for each observation using equation $y_{model} = a + bx$

F value (Table 3): F value tells us whether regression model can predict statistically significantly the dependent variable.

Step 1: Calculate $SS_{residual}$ -It measure the variance in a data set not explained by the regression equation.

Step 2: $df_{residual} = Number\ of\ observations - Number\ of\ parameters$ (here 2 parameters a, x)

Step 3: Calculate Mean residual SS

$$MS_{residual} = \frac{SS_{residual}}{df_{residual}}$$

Step 4: Calculate $SS_{regression}$

Step 5: $df_{regression} = Number\ of\ variables\ being\ studied$

Step 6: Calculate Mean regression SS $MS_{regression} = \frac{SS_{regression}}{df_{regression}}$

Step 7: Calculate F where $F = \frac{MS_{regression}}{MS_{residual}}$

Step 8: Compare calculated F value with table value

Table 3: ANOVA and Regression Procedure

	Df	SS	MS=SS/df	F	Sig.of F
Regression					
Residual					
Total					

Standard error of the estimate/residuals: Average deviation of unexplained variance and obtained by square root of $MS_{residual}$. It is the average distance of observed values from regression line.

R^2 and adjusted R^2: Amount of variance in the outcome that can be explained by the independent variables. Adjusted R^2 is more accurate in this respect. If R^2 is 0.69, it means 69% of the variability can be explained by the independent variables.

$$R^2 = 1 - \left(\frac{SS_{residual}}{SS_{total}}\right),\ Adjusted\ R^2 = 1 - \left(\frac{SS_{residual}}{df_{residual}} \times \frac{df_{total}}{SS_{total}}\right)$$

Using excel function, RSQ we can find out R^2 value.

Significance and CI of Regression coefficient and Slope
Calculation of coefficient is tricky in Logistic regression. IV in both types of regression may be qualitative or quantitative or both.

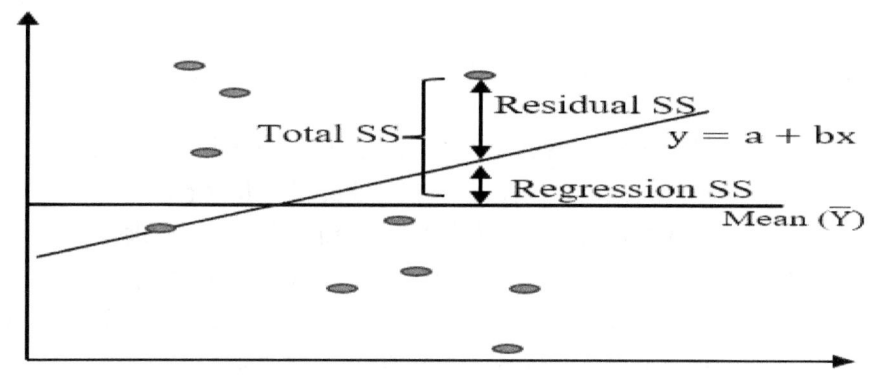

Image 2: Linear Regression Model

Types of Regression

Depends upon the nature of Dependent Variable (Flow Chart 1).

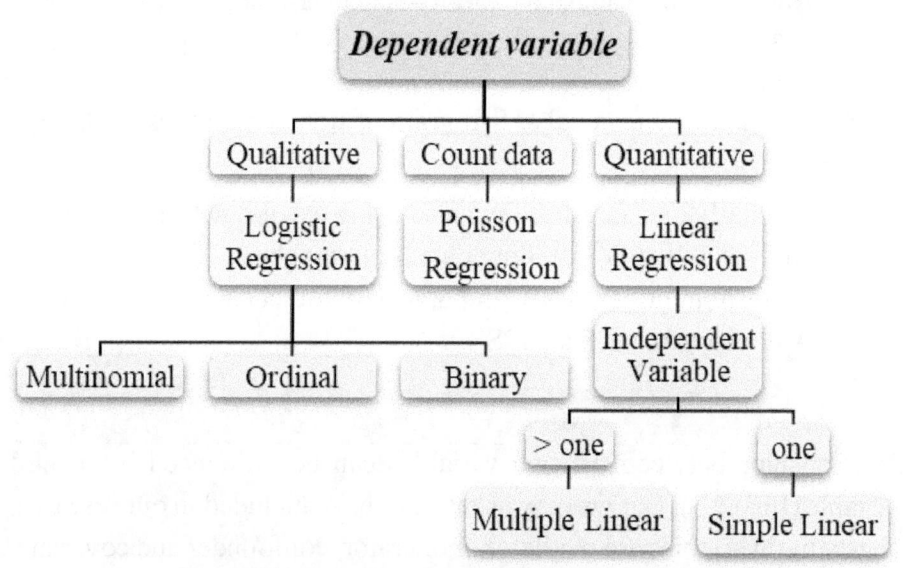

Flow Chart 1: Types of Regression Analysis

Assumptions of Regression

Assumptions of Simple Linear Regression
- Both variables are continuous

- ❖ Linear relationship between DV and IV
- ❖ Residuals normally distributed
- ❖ Homoscedasticity
- ❖ Independence of observations
- ❖ No outlier

Assumptions of Multiple Linear Regression
- ❖ Linear relationship
  - ➢ IV collectively related to DV-Standardized residuals against unstandardized predicted values plot
  - ➢ Each IV is related linearly with DV-partial plots
- ❖ Correlation between residuals- Durbin-Watson statistics
- ❖ Homoscedasticity (equal residual variances)- Standardized residual (Y-axis) against standardized predicted (X-axis)
- ❖ Absence of multicollinearity –when two or more IVs are highly correlated with each other. How to detect?
  None of the IVs have r >0.7, VIF >10 or Tolerance< 0.1
- ❖ Absence of unusual points- Outlier-Standardized residuals >±3/Leverage points- >0.5 dangerous /Influential points- Cook's distance < 1
- ❖ Normality of residuals-Histogram of standardized residuals

Where and How?
- ✓ Manually in excel sheet and also using excel function. Go to data analysis tab after installing data tool kit pack.
- ✓ Perform in https://www.graphpad.com/quickcalcs/
- ✓ Any software such as SPSS

Third Variable

Relationships between the two variables can be influenced by a third variable (Image 3). But we may or may not have included in our research. These third variables are mediator, moderator, confounder and covariate. Mediators and moderators lie on causal pathway whereas confounders and covariates do not lie on causal pathway.

Mediators act as connecting link between the intervention and the outcome of interest. First IV/predictor1 variable has significant effect (significant regression coefficient β) on IV/outcome variable. Second

IV/predictor 2 has also significant effect on outcome variable. Now if we include second IV in the linear regression analysis, effect of first IV becomes insignificant but effect of second IV on outcome variable remains significant. Then second IV/predictor 2 is known as mediator.

Moderators influence relationship between the intervention and the outcome either through direct effect on the outcome, or by interacting with the predictors. Moderators change direction and magnitude (increase/decrease/ negate) of effect on outcome variable (interaction effect). Moderators are also known as effect modifiers.

Confounders are related to both predictors and the outcome, but do not lie on causal pathway. Notice the direction of arrows in confounder and mediator (Both are related to IV and outcome). Moderator and confounder have already been discussed.

Covariates explain a part of the variances in the outcome variable and are not influenced by the predictors. Covariates do not affect the relationship between the predictor variable and the outcome variable. Including covariates in regression analysis, we can find their contribution on outcome.

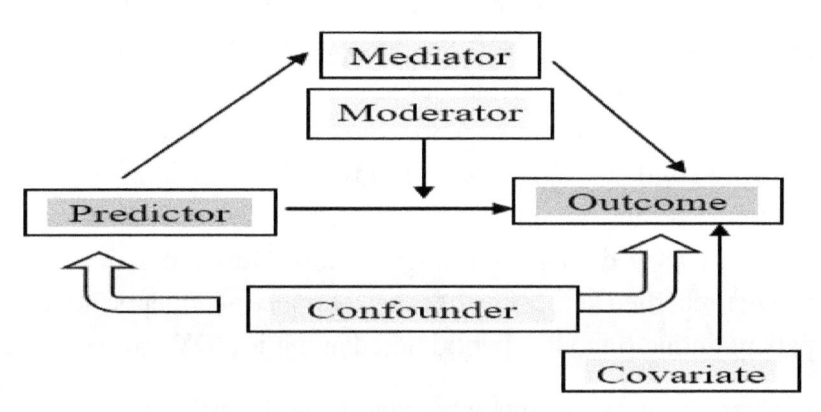

Image 3: Third Variable

Biostatistics in Health Research

Section 2.2: Poisson Regression

In this regression technique, dependent variable (DV) is count of occurrence of an event in a fixed time period. Here, expected count of the event (logarithmic form) is modelled with linear combination of predictors. Mathematically it is expressed as

$log(Y) = \beta_0 + \beta_1 P_1 + \beta_2 P_2 + \beta_3 P_3$ where Y is the **expected** count, β_1, β_2, β_3 are coefficients signifying effects of predictors (P) and P1, P2, P3 are the values of predictors for particular event. For better understanding, we will have to exponentiate the logarithmic form.

Assumptions
- Count data follows Poisson distribution
- $Mean = Variance$
- Occurrence of one event should not influence another event
- There should be linear relationship between logarithm of expected count with the predictors Negative Binomial Regression can be used if there is violation of assumptions.

Applications

Mortality rates following intervention, Rate of hospital acquired pneumonia, Number of seizures following interventions in clinical trial etc. can be modelled with various predictors using this type of regression.

Problem 1: A new antiepileptic drug is being tested for its efficacy compared with a standard drug. Study period 6 months. Participants are randomized into two groups. One group receives new drug and other receives standard drug. Neurological score, Duration of disease, Age and Gender recorded at the time of entry. Number of epileptic attacks in each patient during 6 months period noted and it is a DV (count data).

Problem 2: Sixty patients who have recently suffered from myocardial infarction are being recruited in a study. Researcher is interested to explore the role of age, comorbid conditions, gender, smoking status. Duration of the study 2 years. Number of attack/s (Count data) during the study period for each participant noted.

Section 2.3: Binomial Logistic Regression

Understanding Logistic Regression

This type of regression analysis predicts probability of an observation which falls into one of two categories of DV (binary). Analysis is based on maximum likelihood estimation (MLE) method whereas linear regression is based on ordinary least square (OLS) method. Binomial logistic regression involves at least two IV which may be categorical or continuous.

Assumptions of Binomial Logistic Regression
- Dependent variable is binary
- There should be no multicollinearity among predictors
- Linear relationship between the predictors (continuous) and the logit form of dependent variable.
- No significant outlier
- Adequate sample size usually 10-20 per predictor

Regression Procedure

Regression equation is expressed in the form of

$$Log(\frac{P}{1-P}) = \alpha + \beta_1 X_1 + \beta_2 X_2 + \cdots + \beta_n X_n$$

$Log\left(\frac{P}{1-P}\right)$ is known as logit function. P is the probability of an event occurring whereas 1-P represents event not occurring.

P/(1-P) is called odds. If we take anti log, equation becomes $\frac{P}{1-P} = e^{\alpha+\beta X}$. Thus, $P = e^{\alpha+\beta X}/(1 + e^{\alpha+\beta X})$. After deriving regression coefficients, we can easily calculate the probability of an event occurring. We may do it in excel with Solver. Remember, α is intercept and β is regression coefficient.

Interpretation

Analysis involves two steps: Initially model is described when only intercept is present. Then the model includes predictors and compares the model fit and significance of predictors.

Skills of Reporting Output

Overall Model Fit

Judged usually by Chi-square goodness of fit, -2 loglikelihood ratio and Hosmer-Lemeshow test. Last one examines how poor the model is in predicting, so it should not be significant.

Variance Explained in the Model

Cox & Snell R^2 and Nagalkerke R^2 values are reported to calculate variance explained by the model. R^2 is inappropriate here.

Significance of Predictors

Wald statistic and OR with 95% CI are reported for contribution of predictors. Here value of regression coefficient β states change in Log odds of the dependent variable per unit change in coefficient and this is very difficult to understand. Exp(B) overcome this problem and expresses in terms of OR.

Predictive Accuracy of Logistic Model

Classification Table (Table 4)

Here dichotomous data are classified with a cut-off value of 0.5. Value greater than 0.5 means event occurring. All these are presented in 2*2 table and we can find out what percentages are correctly classified. We may also calculate sensitivity, specificity, Positive Predictive Value (PPV) and Negative Predictive Value (NPV). Higher values are in favor of greater predictivity.

Receiver Operating Characteristic Curve (ROC)

Another important way of reporting predictive capacity is to construct Receiver Operating Characteristic Curve (ROC) with the help of scatterplot of sensitivity and one minus specificity calculated from classification table. Here series of 2*2 tables are prepared as we are now setting range of cut off values instead of 0.5. Area under ROC represents model fit. Area more than 0.5 to 1 favors model fit.

Validation of Model (External Validity)

Examining new data from same population or similar population.

Table 4: Classification Table in Logistic Regression Model

Observed	Predicted Event (1)	Predicted No Event (0)	Total
Event (1)	a	b	a + b
No Events (0)	c	d	c + d
Total	a + c	b + d	a + b + c + d

Advantages of Logistic Regression

Logistic regression does not require following assumptions:
- Linearity of relationship between the DV and IV
- Normality of the error distribution
- Homoscedasticity of the errors

Error/Error Term/Residual

Error refers difference between the observed values and the true values of population. It is a general term. This may occur due to measurement, sampling method, and during prediction as in regression analysis. Error in prediction during regression analysis is also known as residual and is based on sample. In true sense, residual means difference between observed value of an individual in a sample and predicted value from regression analysis based on sample. Thus, error is involved when we consider population (true model) and residual reflects sample (estimated model). Difference between error and 'error term' is error is a general term whereas latter represents specific component of outcome variable which is not explained by the model. In summary, error and residual refers to population deviation and sample deviation respectively.

Let us take an example. Suppose, the mean weight in young population 20-40 year is 50 kg, and now you have chosen randomly one person whose weight is 52, error becomes 2. Now, you collect random sample of 10 (say) persons and mean weight in this sample is 54 kg. If you try to find out difference between sample mean (54) and weight of each person in the sample then you are actually considering residual. So, to conclude difference between weight of each individual in sample and population mean is an error, whereas difference between weight of each individual in sample and sample mean is a residual.

Biostatistics in Health Research

Section 2. 3: Probit Regression Analysis

Probit analysis method is preferred method of studying the dose response relationship. Dose response relationship may be graded or quantal response. In case of quantal response, outcome is binary in nature. In pharmacology, quantal type of dose response relationship is frequently used in toxicity studies such as LD50 estimation. Probit is simply probability unit where percentages are transformed. In toxicity studies, different doses are used in groups of animals and mortality percentages are calculated. Regression analysis is then carried out to estimate LD50 value rather than using DRC.

Skill Development in Probit Regression

Step 1: Number of animals in each group determined.
Step 2: Dose of the drug converted into log dose
Step 3: Calculating mortality and its percentages
Step 4: Probit value for each group corresponding to mortality % (Probit table)
Step 5: Run regression analysis using software or manually taking log dose as independent variable and probit as dependent variable. From here, we find out intercept (a) and regression coefficient beta. Then we form an equation as $Probit = a + (b \times \log dose)$
Step 6: Probit 5 equals 50% mortality, we put a, b and 5 in the equation to find log dose which gives concentration of drug (after taking antilog) that kills 50% of the animal i.e., LD50.

Probit regression analysis with the help of excel is discussed below

From image 5, we find $Y = 2.736X + 1.0523$. So, $X = \frac{(Y - 1.0523)}{2.736}$

As, Y represents 50% death i.e., Probit 5, we will replace Y with 5. Then $X = 1.443$. As, X represents Log10 dose conc., take antilog and we get $X = 27.725$. This is LC50 that kills 50% of animal.

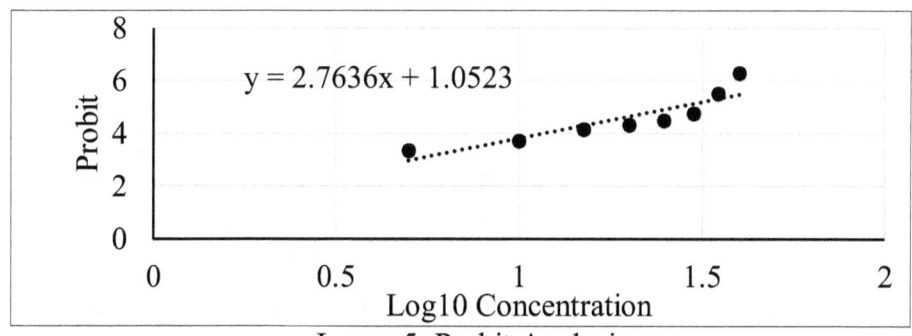

Image 5: Probit Analysis

Table 5: Observation Table for LC50 Study

Drug Conc	Log10 Conc	No Exposed	No Death	% of Death	Probit Value (Finney Table, 1952)
5	0.69	20	1	5	3.36
10	1	20	2	10	3.72
15	1.17	20	4	20	4.16
20	1.30	20	5	25	4.33
25	1.39	20	6	30	4.48
30	1.48	20	8	40	4.75
35	1.54	20	14	70	5.52
40	1.60	20	18	90	6.28

Probit

Quantal type of dose response relationship is frequently used in toxicity studies such as LD50 estimation. In toxicity studies, different doses are used in groups of animals and mortality percentages are calculated and then with the help of formula for correction factor, 0% and 100% mortality are corrected. Probit is calculated on this corrected percentage. This transformed percentages are nothing but 5 plus standard normal deviate of %. Probit value is readily available on Finney's table. Probit 5 means 50% mortality. If we plot probit against log doses, we get a straight line and from there we can easily find out LD50. Log dose corresponding to Probit 5 gives us LD50.

Chapter 9: Bias in Medical Research

Section 1: Bias

Selection Bias

Bias is a process that tend to produce results that depart systematically from true value (Murphy, 1976). There are mainly three types:

Selection Bias

It happens during selection procedures of subjects in both observational and experimental study. Selecting exposed cases through surveillance when there is systematic notification of cases or diagnosing and screening more of the exposed subject results in selection bias. Inclusion of prevalent cases in case control study also carries risk of survival bias.

Types of Selection Bias

Survival Bias- Seen in cases of case control study where prevalent cases rather than incident cases are selected.

Berkson's Bias- it occurs when sample is not selected from general population but from a subpopulation. It was first described by Joseph Berkson in 1946. Both the exposure and disease under study affect the selection. As for example, if cases and control both taken from hospital population, rather than community, it may occur.

Bias due to Nonresponse / Lost to Follow up- When subjects are followed up over a long period as in longitudinal study (cohort and experimental study).

Volunteer Bias- Sampling method involves self-selected members and hence not representative of population. Increasing effort to volunteer in the study along with confidentiality is very important steps for prevention of such type of bias.

Dealing with Selection Bias

Designing stage -Seen in case-control study commonly. Select incident cases and not prevalent cases because prevalent cases may result in survival bias. To use population base design rather than hospital base design, such that the cases and controls are actually selected from the community or the population from where cases come. Eligible criteria, diagnostic procedures and the intensity of surveillance will be same in order to identify cases and controls. Don't select cases /controls based on particular exposure history.

Data collection stage-We should ensure to minimize loss. There may be loss to follow-up where follow –up is over a long period as in cohort study. In that case, we should keep record of all those loss cases including their base line information for analysis in future.

Analysis stage-Compare responders/non-dropouts versus non-responders/dropouts with respect to baseline characteristics. Sensitivity analysis is also helpful to assess direction and magnitude.

Information Bias

Information bias (Measurement bias / Observer bias) occurs when we measure the characteristics of study participants such as exposures, outcomes and other variables that may influence exposures and outcome. So, we should measure it accurately and to be representative one. Information bias in epidemiological study-Both case control study and cohort study are prone to this while taking measurements. Investigator collecting information may support expected conclusion. Biases may occur from subjects distorting the fact.

Types of Information Bias

Recall bias –Seen in case control study where cases recall more exposure history than control. More exposure data is available in cases than controls.

Ascertainment /assessment bias (detection bias or surveillance bias) - occurs when more intense surveillance for outcomes among exposed individuals or differential collection of outcomes.

Prevarication-Systematic distortion of truth by study participants

Dealing with Information Bias

To prevent such biases, detailed measurement protocols, operational definition of variables, training of staffs are essential. Data should be clean before analysis. Blinding and concealment of allocation is efficient method of preventing bias in experimental studies.

Confounding Bias

Confounding is the biggest threat to validity in any epidemiological study. Sometime the effect of exposure / risk factor on outcome variable is distorted due to association of a third variable which is not relevant under study. This third variable is associated with both exposure and outcome and is unequally distributed within exposure and non- exposure groups being compared in the study. A confounder is not in the causal pathway as an intermediate step from exposure to outcome. Details have been discussed in Chapter 4.

Dealing Confounding Bias (Table 1)

Table 1: Dealing Confounding Bias

Stage	Observational Study	Experimental Study
Design	Restriction/ Matching	Restriction/ Matching/ Randomization
Analysis	Stratification/Multivariate	Stratification /Multivariate

Example 1: In a study to find association between coffee drinking and heart attack, cigarette smoking may be a confounding variable as smoking is associated with heart attack and smoking is more in coffee drinkers.

Example 2: Study of association between smoking and lung cancer where age can be a confounding variable as older person more likely to smoke and more chances to develop cancer. Thus, age is related to both exposure (smoking) and outcome (lung cancer).

Example 3: Relationship between obesity and heart disease where age may be confounding variable. Obesity may be more likely in higher age group and heart disease is more likely in old age.

Example 4: Association between birth order and Down syndrome is confounded by maternal age. [Stark CR, Mantel N. Effects of maternal age and birth order on the risk of mongolism and leukemia. Journal of the National Cancer Institute. 1966 Nov 1;37(5):687-98.)]

Section 2: Statistical Errors (Flow Chart)

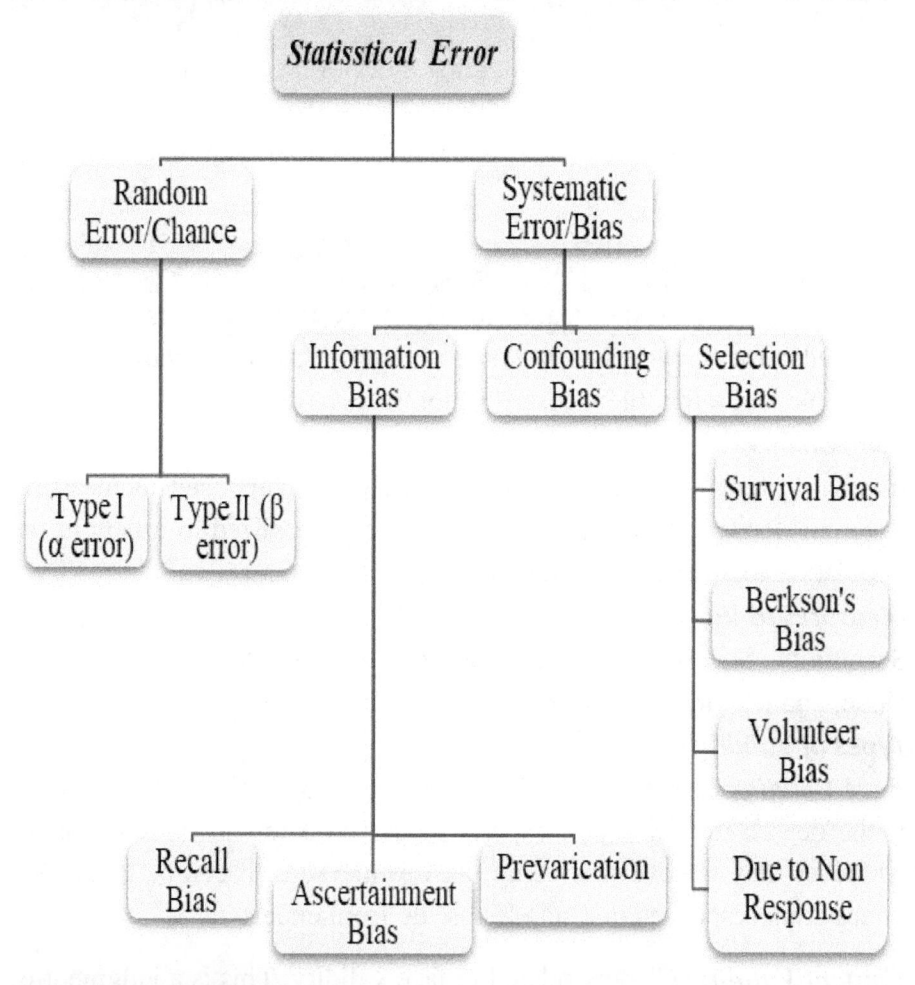

```
                        Statisstical Error
                        ┌───────┴───────┐
                  Random                Systematic
                Error/Chance             Error/Bias
                    │         ┌─────────────┼─────────────┐
                    │    Information    Confounding    Selection
                    │       Bias            Bias          Bias
                    │                                      ├── Survival Bias
            ┌───────┴───────┐                              │
         Type I         Type II (β                         ├── Berkson's Bias
        (α error)        error)                            │
                                                           ├── Volunteer Bias
                                                           │
              Recall    Ascertainment    Prevarication     └── Due to Non
               Bias         Bias                              Response
```

Take Home Messages

- ❖ *Biases can occur in all epidemiological studies*
- ❖ *Biases can occur during all stages of the study*
- ❖ *Biases threaten both the internal and external validity*
- ❖ *Some biases cannot be avoided; we should be aware of this and report it as limitations of the study at the end.*

Chapter 10: Evaluation of a Test or Tool

Section 1: Validity and Reliability

Two things are essential for evaluating a test or measurement tool
- Validity (Accuracy)
- Reliability (Precision, Repeatability, Reproducibility, Internal Consistency)

Validity

Validity of a test is the degree to which the test measures what it is intended to measure. Reliability does not imply validity. A valid measure is reliable, but a reliable measure is not necessarily valid.

Components

Internal-Extent to which it measures what it is supposed to measure. External- How well results of a test can be generalized to others in the population for which it was developed.

Measures of Validity

Sensitivity, Specificity, Positive predictive value, Negative predictive value, and LR (measurements binary).

Types of Validity

Face Validity: It is the subjective view, means by looking at the item. It is the degree to which non-experts perceived a test to be relevant for whatever they believe it is being used to measure. It can be quantified after taking responses in a standard scale from experts.

Content Validity: Closely related to face validity. This is a judgment of whether the conceptual definition has been appropriately translated into operational definition. For instance, if we want to develop a composite scale to measure satisfaction with medical care, then the scale should include all important features of medical care.

It is estimated by a group of experts in the particular field. All the items on the tool are assessed separately and given a score on a 3-point or 4-point Likert scale. Content Validity Index (CVI) is computed for each item as the number of experts judging the item as relevant or not relevant and then divided by the total number of experts in the team.

Construct Validity: It is concerned with what quality does a test measure. It is evaluated by demonstrating that certain explanatory construct (domain) accounts for some degree of performance on the test. For example, a measure of job satisfaction might be compared with the information on what the subjects do, since it is reasonable to predict some degree of association. It can be estimated by:
- Internal Consistency - It verifies that a particular item or section measures the same characteristic individually that the test as a whole measure.
- Factor Analysis

Criterion Validity: It is the degree to which a test result matches up with the other known measures of the characteristics (gold standard). There are 2 types:

Concurrent Validity - Result of a new indicator is compared with another established indicator for the same characteristics at the same time. For example, if we want to develop a new scale to assess anxiety, then it is administered at the same time with some established scale. If the results are similar, then the new scale has criterion validity.

Predictive Validity - Degree to which a test predicts results of a variable to be measured at some future point of time. For example, for police selection test, applicants who scored low on the test (but passed and hired) had more disciplinary citations in their records a year later than the persons who scored high on the test. The test has a predictive validity in that it predicts a subsequent behavior.

Convergent and Discriminant Validity: It is based on a comparison with other measures of the same variable. If it is uncertain whether the other measure is superior to the one being checked, then convergent validity is checked rather than criterion validity. A new tool of mental health would be expected to show a strong correlation with other mental health measures. This new tool would not be expected to show a strong correlation with a standard tool.

Reliability

It is the extent to which the measurements of a test remain consistent when repeated on the same subjects under identical conditions. It is to be noted that there are subtle differences between repeatability and reproducibility. Where Validity is related with systematic error or bias, reliability is concerned with random error.

Types of Reliability
- Inter-rater reliability: Degree to which different observers give consistent results of the same measurement.
- Test–Re-test reliability: Consistency of results on two separate occasions.
- Parallel–Forms reliability: Consistency of results of two parallel forms of same test conducted in the same way.
- Internal Consistency reliability: Consistency of results across items within a test

Estimation of Reliability

There are mainly three methods: Test - retest method, Split-half method and Cronbach's alpha (α). Here I shall focus on Cronbach's alpha.

Cronbach's Alpha

Suppose a set of questions/items in an instrument /scale measure a particular characteristic. Cronbach's alpha says whether the items measure the same concept reliably. In contrast, validity refers to it measures what it is meant to measure.

Assumptions of Cronbach's alpha
- All items should measure the same concept
- All items share variances equally for the concept
- Linear relationship between items
- Items should have equal error variance (not explained by true score)
- Both Qualitative and Quantitative data can be analysed

Application
Testing reliability/consistency of a Questionnaire/Instrument/Scale

Section 2: Frequently Asked Questions

1. What do you mean by Precision?

Precision/Reliability/Internal consistency: Closeness of an estimate to the true population parameter. Alternatively representing degree to which measured values are close to each other. In true sense, results may be precise if we are getting similar findings each time the study is done. Lack of precision is referred to as random error. If repeated measurements of an item in the same subjects under identical conditions produce identical results, our inference is measurement is reliable.

Validity- Validity means does it measure what it is supposed to measure the true value. Lack of validity results in Bias.

Accuracy- Ability of a measurement to be correct on the average and though includes both precision and validity, accuracy truly states the concepts of systematic error or bias. In statistics, reliability or precision is measured using random error and validity by bias. We refer the term validity as a qualitative equivalent of accuracy. In validity, we mean how well a study outcome or measurement reflects a phenomenon of interest i.e we are adding qualitative dimensions or flavors to the term accuracy.

2. What are the sources of random error?
   - Variation in observer
   - Variation in instrument and environment
   - Subject variation which is very important

3. How to reduce random error or increase precision?
   - Operational guidelines of measurements of variables
   - Training of research team
   - High quality instruments and automated instruments
   - Taking repeated measurements at least three times and taking average of these. Most practical way to reduce random error is to increase sample size.

4. How will you measure precision?
   - Qualitative –Kappa statistics or percent agreement
   - Quantitative- Coefficient of variation and Bland –Altman plot

6. How to reduce systematic or bias and thus increase accuracy?

Measures are same as in case of precision, study design is very important.

Blinding may enhance accuracy. Appropriate design of the study is the practical way to prevent bias. Increasing sample size has no effect.

7. How will you assess accuracy?

Qualitative-Sensitivity, Specificity, PPV, NPV (compare the measurements with gold standard which is taken as best representative of measurement).
Quantitative- Mean difference

8. Reproducibility/Replication-In repeatability, we take repeated measurements of the same item during same experimental runs. Doing experiment multiple times by the researcher is reproducibility.

9. Discuss different types of validity? Write measures of validity?

10. What is questionnaire? What are the different types?

It is a research instrument that contains a series of standard question for collecting study related information from respondents. It is of two types- Interviewer administered and Self-administered (Flow Chart 1).

11. What are the differences between random and systematic error?

Table 1: Difference between Random error and Systematic Error

Random Error /Chance	Systematic Error /Bias
Distorts results in both direction	Distorts results in one direction
Precision used for assessment	Accuracy used for assessment
Increasing sample size increases precision	Appropriate study design decreases bias

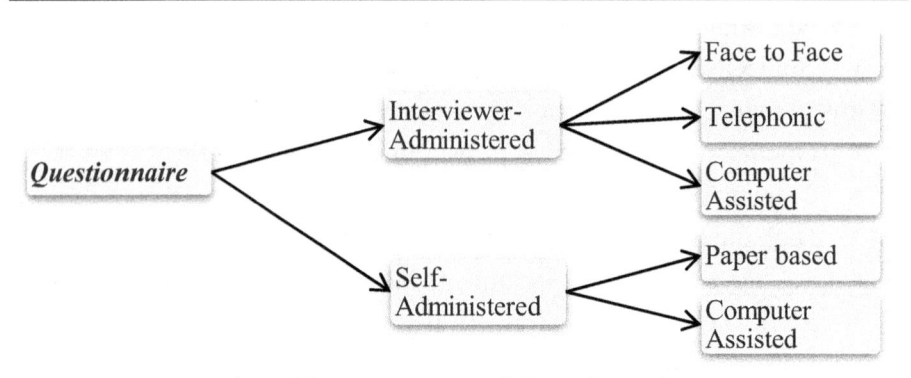

Flow Chart 1: Types of Questionnaires

Chapter 11: Diagnostic Test Study

Section 1: Validity for Binary Data

In assessment of diagnostic test, we require gold standard which is taken as a reference or 100% accurate in diagnosing the condition and the subjects or test material undergo testing in both Diagnostic test which is a new one and gold standard. Two parameters are evaluated: Reliability assessed by calculating kappa coefficient and other is validity measured by sensitivity, specificity, Positive Predictive Value (PPV), Negative Predictive Value (NPV) and Likelihood Ratios (+ and -). For better understanding, we are presenting results of RTPCR and Rapid antigen test for diagnosis of Covid-19 in table 1. RTPCR is taken as gold standard here.

Table 1: Diagnostic Test Evaluation

Rapid Antigen Test	RTPCR	
	Positive	Negative
Positive	TP(a)	FP(b)
Negative	FN(c)	TN(d)

Sensitivity is the ability or probability of detecting those positive cases who really have the disease (as per gold standard) whereas Specificity is the probability or ability of detecting as negative cases who really don't have the disease (as per gold standard).

$$\text{Sensitivity} = \frac{a}{(a+c)} = \frac{TP}{(TP+FN)}, \quad \text{Specificity} = \frac{b}{(b+d)} = \frac{TN}{(TN+FP)}$$

As a clinician, we are not interested in estimating sensitivity/specificity, rather we want to know if a person is positive on new diagnostic agent, what is the actual chance of having disease or if negative, what is the actual chance of not having the disease. To overcome the problem, we calculate the probability if a person is tested positive or negative, what is the chance of it. PPV and NPV give us confidence. There is a problem with those two predictive values as they depend on prevalence of disease. But value of sensitivity and specificity will not change if the test is carried out in any setting.

$$PPV = \frac{a}{(a+b)} = \frac{TP}{(TP+FP)}, \quad NPV = \frac{d}{(c+d)} = \frac{TN}{(FN+TN)}.$$

In high prevalence are PPV is high and in low prevalence area it is low. This has got tremendous impact in clinical settings. By preparing a table described above, it can be shown that in low prevalence area, high positive rate by the new diagnostic test includes huge false positive cases resulting in dangerous consequences. It should further be confirmed and to be repeated on second time even third time on positive cases to overcome this problem where PPV value is improved.

This can be shown with the help of table where repeated positive cases undergo testing with new diagnostic test. This is a real scenario as most of the diagnostic test during their development, validation is carried out in high prevalence area and to impress clinician's sensitivity and specificity with high value which is fixed are commonly marketed but manufacturer do not mention place.

This is very important aspect while evaluating a diagnostic test. This sort of problem when we are doing in low prevalence area can be adjusted by above procedure of repeated testing on positive cases.

When a test has sensitivity, it gives positive results on large number of individuals who don't have the disease i.e. it includes huge number of false positive cases. Positive test results cannot confirm positivity, but negative result says that the subject is not diseased. So, positive cases are confirmed in next step by means of any gold standard. Thus, a test with high sensitivity is an ideal test for initial screening. In a test with high specificity, positive result confirms but negative result does not mean that subject is not diseased as negative results in a test with high specificity includes huge number of false negative cases. This type of test is good for confirmatory testing.

As clinicians are more interested in predictive values, we are not confident about the results because of its dependence on prevalence status. To overcome such problem, we calculate positive and negative likelihood ratio. This ratio combines the information of both sensitivity and specificity and gives more insight about the quality of test and is preferred by researchers while validating.

$$LR(+) = \frac{Sensitivity}{1-Specificity}, \quad LR(-) = \frac{1-Sensitivity}{Specificity}$$

LR (+) tells us the probability of positive result in diseased compared to non-diseased whereas LR (-) gives us probability of negative results in diseased compared to non-diseased. LR (+) 5 means positive results 5 times likely in diseased compared to those who don't have the disease. Thus, we have learnt about various parameters about validity and how they give us confidence. Remember, highly sensitive test gives positive results even in non-diseased (FP). So, negative test results with highly sensitive test almost confirms that the subject is non-diseased. This is the reason why highly sensitive test is used for screening test. If you think of highly specific test, most of becomes negative and few becomes positive. It is almost certain these positive cases are diseased and thus can be used as diagnostic test.

Above method of validation is applicable when results of diagnostic test are recorded in a dichotomous scale but for continuous data, go for ROC (Receiver Operating Characteristic Curve). Measures of Validity has been presented in Flow Chart 1.

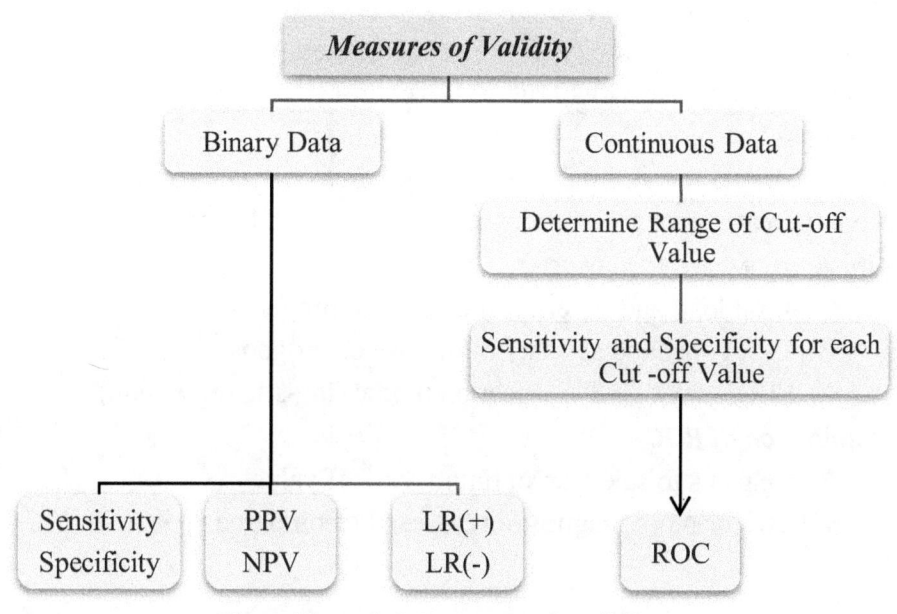

```
                    Measures of Validity
                    /              \
              Binary Data      Continuous Data
                                    |
                          Determine Range of Cut-off Value
                                    |
                          Sensitivity and Specificity for each Cut-off Value
                                    |
   Sensitivity    PPV    LR(+)     ROC
   Specificity    NPV    LR(-)
```

Flow Chart 1: Measures of Validity

Section 2: Validity for Continuous Data

Receiver Operating Characteristic (ROC) Curve

Steps of Construction of ROC (Image 1)
Step 1: Record continuous outcome value of the diagnostic test
Step 2: Put results of gold standard (dichotomous/binary)
Step 3: Decide a cut off value above which disease present or not.
Step 4: Put results of gold standard in 2x2 contingency table
Step 5: Calculate Sensitivity and Specificity
Step 5: In this way, multiple tables prepared for different cut off value, calculate Sensitivity and Specificity for each cut-off value.
Step 6: Prepare a table where each cut off value has sensitivity, specificity and 1-Specificity (At least 3 cut-off values required)
Step 7: Plot 1-Specificity in X axis and Sensitivity in Y axis
Step 8: Join the points and for optimum cut off, we use information of sensitivity and specificity and construct what is called ROC

Description of the Curve
X-axis shows 1-specificity (False positive rate)
Y axis shows Sensitivity (True positive rate)
Diagonal line represents No predictive ability
Area under the curve >0.5 represents predictive/diagnostic ability. Test having greater area is better compared to test with lesser area.

Situations where ROC is used
- Viral load and severity of disease or prognosis
- CRP conc. and severity of disease or prognosis
- Efficiency of a classification model (logistic regression)

Application of ROC
- Helps us to select an optimum cut-off value
- Two or more diagnostic tests can be compared.

Image 1: ROC Curve

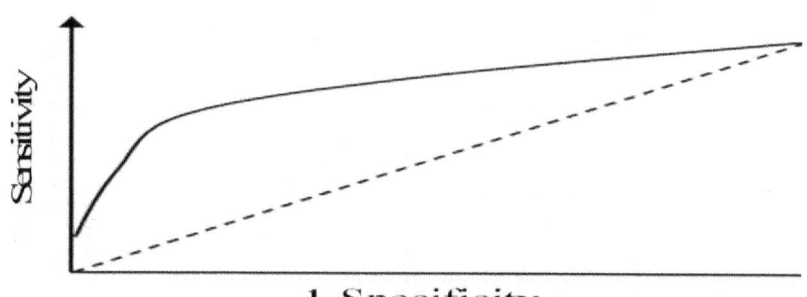

Sensitivity vs *1-Specificity*

Skills on Statistical Calculation

Table 2: Hypothetical Data in Covid 19 Patients

Throat swab	PCR (Gold Standard) Positive	PCR (Gold Standard) Negative	Total
Positive	100(a)	900(b)	1000(a+b)
Negative	20(c)	880(d)	900(c+d)
Total	120(a+c)	1760(b+d)	1900(a+b+c+d)

Here, $a = TP, b = FP, c = FN, d = TN$. Putting all these values, we can calculate the following parameter

$$Sensitivity = \frac{a}{(a+c)} = \frac{TP}{(TP+FN)} = \frac{100}{120} = 0.83$$

$$Specificity = \frac{b}{(b+d)} = \frac{TN}{(TN+FP)} = \frac{900}{1760} = 0.51$$

$$PPV = \frac{a}{(a+b)} = \frac{TP}{(TP+FP)} = \frac{100}{1000} = 0.1$$

$$NPV = \frac{d}{(c+d)} = \frac{TN}{(FN+TN)} = \frac{880}{900} = 0.97$$

$$LR(+) = \frac{Sensitivity}{1-Specificity} = \frac{0.83}{1-0.51} = \frac{0.83}{0.49} = 1.69$$

$$LR(-) = \frac{1-Sensitivity}{Specificity} = \frac{1-0.83}{0.51} = \frac{0.17}{0.51} = 0.33$$

Chapter 12: Measures of Agreement

Section 1: Understanding Agreement

Sometimes we are interested whether the measurements/scores from two or more raters/observers or methods/instruments are similar or not-this represents agreement. Variable may be qualitative or quantitative. Depending on type of measurements and number of observers, types of analysis vary (Flow Chart 1). We will restrict our discussion to Cohen's kappa and Bland-Altman plot.

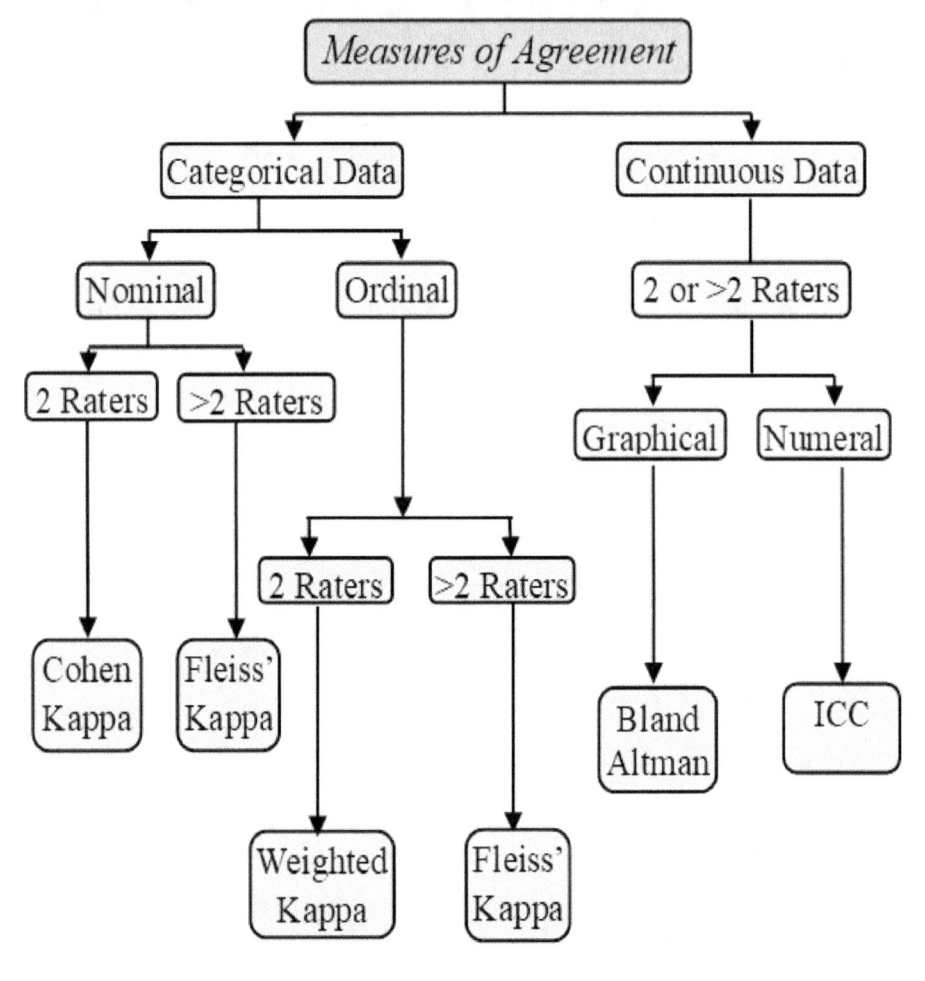

Flow Chart 1: Analysis of Agreement

Section 2: Common Measures of Agreement

Cohen Kappa

It is the level of agreement between two raters for categorical items. Cohen's kappa includes probability of random agreement in calculation and is given by $\kappa = \frac{P_O - P_e}{1 - P_e}$

Where P_O = Observed agreement(relative) between raters
P_e = Probability of random agreement.

Kappa value 0 means equivalent to chance agreement, 1 means perfect agreement and negative value indicates disagreement. Let us take an example. In a mental health screening camp, 50 patients are being categorized by both psychiatrist and general physician into two groups- Functional and Neurological (Table 1).

Table 1: Agreement between Two Raters

		General Physician	
		Functional	Neurological
Psychiatrist	Functional	5	10
	Neurological	9	26

We know, P_O = Observed agreement(relative) between raters, this means persons classified as functional by both raters (here 5) and neurological (here 15) by both raters. Thus, $P_O = \frac{5+26}{50} = 0.62$.

Now, as calculation of Cohen's kappa includes chance/random agreement, we will calculate this in the following way.
Again, P_e=Probability of random agreement
Probability of functional by psychiatrist=15/50=0.3
And by General physician=14/50=0.28
Probability of categorizing as functional by both=0.3 * 0.28
Probability of neurological by both=$\frac{35}{50} * \frac{36}{50}$=0.5
Overall probability of random agreement (P_e)=0.084 + 0.5=0.5
(To understand calculation of random agreement, readers are advised to go through the laws of probability)

We know, $k = Po - Pe/1 - Pe$. Substituting all these values, $k = \frac{0.62-0.5}{1-0.5} = \frac{0.12}{0.5} = 0.2$. Value 0.2 represents slight agreement.

Bland-Altman Plot

This type of plot measures the degree of agreement between two continuous measurements of two methods or scores of two raters. Here, we construct 95% CI of the mean difference between two methods. 95% of the data should lie within 2 SD of the Mean Difference. We can plot the difference as unit, percentage or ratio. Researcher should decide limits of agreement before the study and it depends upon the clinical or biological aspects. This type of analysis cannot be done by estimation of correlation coefficient because of the following reasons:

- ❖ Correlation deals with two different variables whereas this plot requires same variable on two occasions.
- ❖ High correlation does not guarantee agreement
- ❖ Correlation does not involve difference

Assumptions: Differences between two measurements should be normally distributed (Shapiro-Wilk / Kolmogorov-Smirnov test).

Procedure: Bland-Altman plot can easily be presented graphically through excel or any software. It is a scatter plot where X-axis displays averages of two measurements and Y-axis differences between two measurements (Table 2 and Image 1).

Step 1: Col 1 and Col 2 records measurements of two instruments
Step 2: Col 3 shows averages of the two
Step 3: Col 4 shows differences between measurements
Step 4: Calculate Mean of Diff (4.25) and SD of Diff (6.01)
Step 5: Calculate CI=Mean Difference±1.96*SD (16.04, -7.5)
Step 6: In excel, go to scatter plot where X-axis represents averages of the two and Y-axis differences between two measurements
Step 7: Now stepwise, draw three horizontal lines (one for mean difference and other two for upper and lower limits as calculated)
Limits of Agreement=Mean Diff ± 1.96*SD (Diff)

Observations: Look for three things before interpretation: Position of bias line, Scatter around bias line and Trend of differences.

Table 2: BP Recording in Old and New Instrument

Old Machine	New Machine	Average	Difference
110	105	107.5	5
115	113	114	2
132	126	129	6
108	113	110.5	-5
111	111	111	0
117	101	109	16
111	105	108	6
122	118	120	4

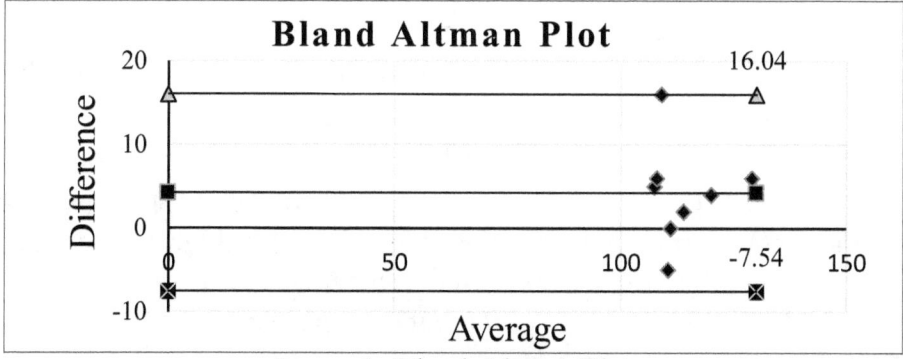

Image 1: Bland-Altman Plot

Proportional Bias in Bland-Altman Plot

When there is increase in average of the two measurements, there is increase or decrease in differences in measurements, then we say that proportional bias exists. It should be detected by inspection of scatter plot. Some statistical procedure such as Regression analysis or correlation coefficient between the measurements are used to quantify proportional bias. Possible causes should be explored in this situation. Logarithmic transformation of the data is essential to stabilize variances before carrying out the procedure. Presence of proportional bias affects reliability and validity of results.

Chapter 13: Survival Analysis

Section 1: Basic Understanding of Survival Analysis

When outcome variable is time to event such as death, injury, heart attack, recurrence, recovery from an illness, withdrawing ventilation, control of loose motion, subsidence of fever etc., we use survival analysis. Survival means probability of remaining free of event of interest for a specific period of time. Survival analysis data are gathered from cohort study or RCT. Information from participant about time to event is not normally distributed. Another disadvantage of this type of data is the presence of censoring. Censoring means incomplete information and this may occur in cases where participant leaves the study for unknown reasons, withdraw consents from the study or left the study area due to some personal problems. Censoring may also occur if the participant does not suffer from the event during the study period. One important term is to be mentioned here is Survival Function at time t given by $S(t) = \dfrac{Number\ of\ patients\ surviving\ after\ time\ t}{Total\ number\ of\ patients}$.

Objectives of Survival Analysis
- ❖ Estimate time to event (entry into the study to occurrence of events)
- ❖ Comparing two or more groups
- ❖ Effect of covariates

Advantages of Survival Analysis
- ❖ Handle non-normal data
- ❖ Incomplete information censored data into the analysis
- ❖ Risk assessment
- ❖ Effect of covariates can be estimate

Analysis

If there is no censoring, we may perform non parametric test such as Mann Whitney U along with reporting of median and inter-quartile range. As time to event data have non normal distribution, parametric test cannot be done. Regression method does not include censoring data. Though several methods are used, Kaplan-Meier method (KM plot) is popular. In this survival curve, Y- axis shows proportion of individuals at risk of an event of interest, and X- axis indicates time. Study period is not divided into interval, survival time is recorded each time subject has an event. More than 50% uncensored observations are required KM plot.

Assumptions of KM Plot
- ❖ Record exactly when the event or censorship occurred
- ❖ Causes of censoring not to be related with event of interest
- ❖ Factors that affect the event of interest should not change during study period such new treatment regimen, new technology for diagnosis.
- ❖ "Similar amount" and similar "patterns" of censorship /group

For comparing two or more groups, log rank test is performed and calculates hazard ratio (similar to odds ratio) and assumes that risk of event of interest remains same throughout the study. Cox regression method includes covariates also time dependent covariates. Equation is given by $h(t) = h_0 e^{\beta_1 X_1 + \beta_2 X_2 \ldots + \beta_k X_k}$, h_0 represents baseline hazard and there involves no covariates. X1, X2…are the covariates and β measure the effect size of the covariate. In Cox regression, there is no intercept which is present in logistic or linear regression. Here, predictors may be categorical and continuous and number of predictors ≥ 2 whereas in Kaplan Meier plot, there is only one categorical predictor.

Biostatistics in Health Research

Section 2: Frequently Asked Questions

1. What is survival? Give example.
2. What is survival function? Write advantages.
3. What is the difference between odds ratio and hazard ratio?
4. Write two assumptions of Cox regression.
5. What are the disadvantages of KM plot?
6. Write five examples where survival plot is appropriate method of analysis.
7. Differentiate between Cox regression, Binary logistic regression, Poisson regression and linear regression. Give example for each.
8. Write down steps of Kaplan Meier plot in excel.
9. Enumerate five important features of Kaplan Meier plot.

Example 1

Out of 200 Scrub typhus patients diagnosed clinically, 85 received Azithromycin and 85 received Doxycycline. Time to remission of fever after introduction of drug was recorded. Four patients lost to follow up and one died in Azithromycin group whereas nine lost to follow up and two died in Doxycycline group. Three patients in first group and one patient in second group had no remission of fever during the study period (5 days). Clinician wants to know whether the difference in defervescence period is due to drug therapy? (KM Plot)

In the above situation, researcher included patients' nutritional status, presence of primary complex and tried to find whether these factors have any contribution for time to remission of fever. Which type of analysis is appropriate here? (Cox Regression)

Chapter 14: Sampling

Section 1: Different Terms Used in Sampling

Basic Terms

Population
Includes all individuals or objects of specific characteristic in a defined area. It may be finite when total number can be counted or may be infinite.

Census and Sample Survey (Table 1)
When we undertake a study, either we take all individuals i.e. complete enumeration (Census) or part of the population is studied (Survey).

Sample
A finite number of units selected from the population.

Unit /Individual
Each member of the population or sample and may be an individual or group of individuals.

Sample Size
Number of units or individuals in the sample.

Sampling
Method of collecting units/individuals in a sample.

Sampling Fraction
Proportion of population that is in the sample which is given by the formula Population size / Sample size.

Sampling Interval
Interval between sampling unit, used in systematic random sampling.

Sampling Error
Difference between estimates obtained in sample and actual value in population. If sample size is increased, error decreases.

Non- sampling Error
Arises at different stages of sampling procedure starting from planning to data analysis and tabulation. Non sampling error is more in census as it lacks proper planning, training of staffs, less involved in in-depth investigation of all members.

Table1: Census and Sampling Survey

Census	Sampling Survey
Enumeration of all units	Part of population taken
No sampling error	Sampling error present
No Standard error	Standard error present
Hypothesis testing not done	Hypothesis testing done
Non-sampling error more	Non-sampling error less
Planning, training of staffs, monitoring, supervision and in-depth investigation not done properly	Highly accurate

Population and Sample (Flow Chart 1)

Target population or Theoretical population or Reference population or Universe – Selected from population of large geographical area on the basis of *Clinical and Demographic* Characteristics. Study population (also known as the accessible population) is the population that is derived from the target population on the basis of *Geographical and Temporal Characteristics* for the smooth conduction of the research. This specific group of people is manageable, much easy to sample for conducting research. Study sample /study subject- selected from accessible population for study and results of study are generalized (external validity) to accessible population and target population.

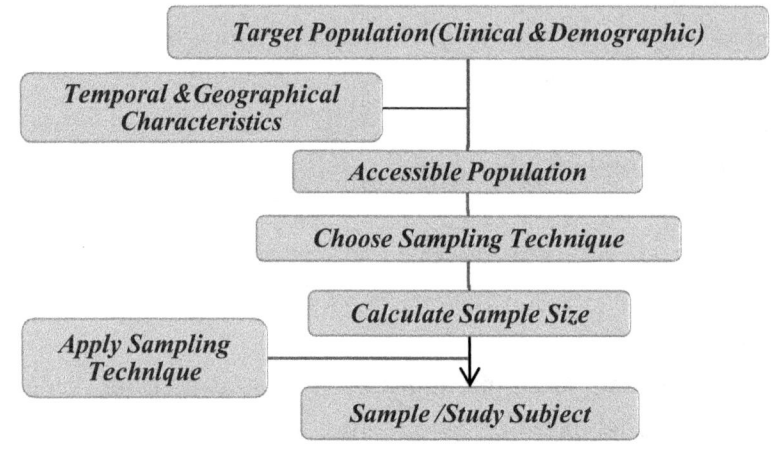

Flow Chart 1: Sample Selection from Population

Section 2: Sampling Technique

Two types –one is probability sampling and another is non probability sampling (Flow chart 2). Probability sampling is governed by laws of chance where each unit in the population has an equal chance of being selected in the sample. Statistical analysis can appropriately be applied in this case and inference can be drawn about population. Different types of sampling procedure and their application with demerits and steps have been discussed in the following section.

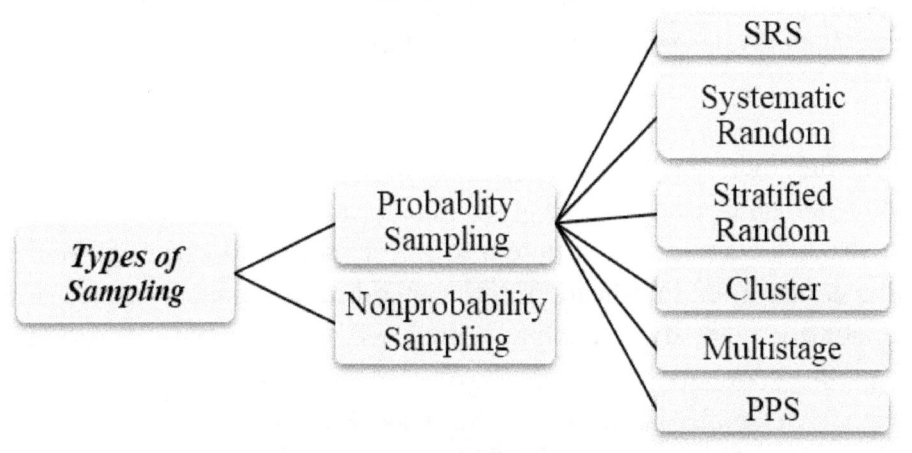

Flow Chart 2: Types of Sampling

Probability Sampling

Simple Random Sampling (SRS)

Here each unit/individual has equal chance of being included in the sample. Done when the sample size is small, homogeneous and selected sampling unit is spread over small area.

Method of randomness
- Lottery method
- Random number table
- Computer generated random number

Steps
Step 1: Determine size of population (sampling frame)
Step 2: Numbering all units
Step 3: Decide sample size

Step 4: Select individuals using any of the above method
Merits: Units in the population have an equal and independent chance of being selected. Simple and easy to perform.
Demerits: Sampling frame must be prepared or should be ready before the procedure.
- Difficult in case of large sample size
- Also, difficult when sample units are dispersed over large area.
- Sample may not always be representative of population

Application: Selecting suppose 20 students out of 42 in a school to estimate prevalence of hookworm infestation through stool test.

Systematic Random Sampling

Selecting individuals/units at regular interval from the sampling frame after first unit being selected at random. This method is usually applied at the last stage or in the intermediate steps of multistage sampling. Sometimes after stratification, this method of sampling is carried out. Systematic method of sampling is preferred when sample is large. Full sampling frame preparation is not essential always, knowledge of total frame is essential as in hospital settings where after fixing first unit, patient attending clinic is recruited at regular interval depending upon the sampling interval.

Method: First unit at random then other members at regular interval.
Step 1: Determine size of population (sampling frame), Suppose 20
Step 2: Numbering all units serially based on some characteristic
Step 3: Decide sample size, Suppose 5
Step 4: Calculate sampling interval, here 20/5=4
Step 5: Select one member randomly from first 4 members. This is the first unit of sample. Say it is 3, so third person is the first unit.
Step 6: Now units in sample have following serial number: 3,6,9,12,15
Merits: Can be conveniently used in large sample
Demerits: Only the starting point is random, in true sense it is not random sample. If there is trend, may not be appropriate method
Application: Selecting OPD patients with stage 2 hypertension for testing efficacy of lisinopril over amlodipine.

Probability Proportional to Size (PPS)

Here probability of selecting a sample unit is proportional to its population size. This type of sampling method is highly helpful where sampling units vary considerably in size to make a highly representative of sampling units of all sizes.

Suppose we want to select 3 schools from a district and then we take 10 students from each school. If we take random sample of schools from the district, we will get biased towards the selection of schools because number of students vary considerably from school to school. Probability of a school with small number of students being selected is less than large sized school. Instead of applying SRS, we use PPS method to avoid such selection bias. In above example, selection of schools from the district and not the selection of students from the school will be based on PPS. Basically, systematic random sampling is applied to the cumulative number of students of the schools.

Steps (Table 2)

Step 1: Arrange schools in ascending number of students (say 5 schools in district)
Step 2: Make a separate column to the right for cumulative number
Step 3: Calculate total cumulative students at all school (here 75)
Step 4: Decide No of schools to be selected (here 3)
Step 5: Find sampling interval = Step 3/Step 4 = 75/3 = 25
Step 6: Select a random number between 1 and 25 (say is 14)
Step 7: Now draw systematic random sampling in PPS sampling (14, 14+25, 14+25+25, i.e., PPS includes 14, 39, 64)

Table 2: PPS through Systematic Random Sampling

School	Number of Students	Cumulative Number	PPS
1	10	10	
2	12	22	14
3	15	37	
4	18	55	39
5	20	75	64

Demerits: Size of each sampling unit in population is to be known.
Application: Vaccination coverage in a community

Stratified Sampling

When population is not homogeneous, it is classified into homogenous groups called strata from where we select sample units either through SRS or systematic random sampling. Number of sample units to be selected from each stratum must be proportional to the size of the stratum. Stratification may be done on the basis of any characteristic (age, sex, income etc.) which a researcher thinks necessary for study.

Merits: Enhances representativeness, more accurate and sampling error is reduced.

Demerits: Takes more time to get units stratum wise, costly and more difficult to obtain proportionality.

Cluster Sampling

When sampling procedure involves large area where sampling frame that includes every unit is difficult or impossible to construct or costly and requires more time, we divide the area into small area known as clusters. Sometimes natural grouping exists such as schools, hospital, Factory and geographical areas etc. After formation of clusters, required number of clusters is taken using SRS or systematic random sampling or PPS. The units or individuals within the clusters should be as homogeneous as possible. Table 3 shows differences between Stratified and Cluster sampling

Merits
- No list of units or sampling frame is required
- Less cost and less travel expenses
- When large population are studied

Demerits
- High sampling error and is difficult to measure
- To achieve same precision as in SRS, more units are to be included.
- Design effect is considered while calculating sample size. This has been discussed at the end of this chapter.

Application: Vaccination coverage in UIP

Table 3: Differences between stratified and cluster sampling

Stratified Sampling	Cluster Sampling
Population is divided into few strata	Population is divided into many clusters
Sample units drawn from each	Sample units drawn from few
Stratum specific estimate possible	Cluster wise estimate not possible
Main objective is cost reduction	Increase precision

Multi-stage Sampling

Carried out in two or more stages where sampling frame, sampling units, number of selected units and sampling procedure may differ in various stages. It is mainly adopted when large region is involved (district, state or even a country). In each stage, decide sampling unit and its number to be selected and then construct sampling frame and finally adopt appropriate sampling procedure.

Application: While carrying out nutritional status in a district through household survey, households should be representative.

Stage 1: Sampling unit is block; sampling frame is lists of blocks, Sampling method through which specified number of blocks are selected may be stratified/PPS/systematic/cluster.

Stage 2: Sampling unit is village; sampling frame is lists of villages, sampling method through which specified numbers of villages are selected may be PPS/systematic.

Stage 3: Sampling unit is household; sampling frame is lists of households, sampling method through which specified numbers of villages are selected may be SRS/systematic.

Merits: When large area involved, can be easily conducted with less cost in a more efficient way and variability is reduced.

Which Sampling Procedure?

Usually, method of choice is SRS. If sample size is small and sampling frame available go for SRS. When sample size is large and sampling frame available (only knowledge of sampling frame is required) perform systematic random sampling. In cases of nonavailability of sampling frame where large, dispersed area is involved and adequate representation is important, situations are handled with multiple types of procedure. For adequate representation, stratification is required for making homogeneous strata and subsequently stratified sampling.

Cluster method of sampling is applicable for situation involving large geographical region and natural groupings present or divided into clusters. Multiple procedures may be done in a particular problem and is frequently seen in practice.

Non-probability Sampling

Overview of Non-probability Sampling

Non-probability sampling method less likely produces representative and accurate sample. Samples are taken as per availability and in non-random fashion. Sample units are selected based on accessibility, convenience, judgment and purpose.

When is it used?
- When there is limited time, less budget and manpower
- When sampling frame is difficult to construct
- Objective of research is not to draw conclusion about population but exploratory in nature. Trying to find reasons behind a particular phenomenon. To study in-depth of a certain behaviour. If no research so far conducted, in the initial phase go for qualitative research where this type of sampling method is used to know the fact.

Merits and demerits: This type of sampling method does not provide probability as selection is not at random but by choice and depends upon various factors specifically accessibility. Therefore, it is not amenable to statistical tests though averages and dispersion can be calculated. Results cannot be generalized. In large samples, though non-random, it may be considered adequate for valid inferences. Qualitative research mostly uses this type of sampling method. Because of less time and budget, this can be quickly performed

Types of Non-probability Sampling

Convenience Sampling

Anybody who is likely to be suitable for the study (after interviewing) are included and here investigator takes sample while walking on street, in public places or in any gathering and process continues till required number collected.

Snowball Sampling

In case of rare or sensitive events being studied, we adopt this method. Subjects are utilized to identify a greater number of cases rather than detailed survey. Thus, reduces the cost and saves time. Due to sensitive nature of subject matter, cases do not come, and we cannot construct sampling frame. Studying prevalence of AIDS or STD, we can trace others with the help of respondent.

Quota Sampling

In the first step, we stratify the population of interest and then depending upon investigators choice, subjects are included in non-random fashion within each stratum till predetermined adequate number (quota) is completed in them.

Area Sampling

Sampling frame is constructed using maps rather than lists or registers. Then area is divided into small areas using maps and from there units are selected using SRS or systematic random sampling.

Design Effect: Calculation of sample size in most of the cases assumes that Simple Random Sampling (SRS) was used. But it is not always true. Sometimes we use cluster, systemic, stratified or PPS method for participant recruitment. In these situations, due to altered variability actual sample size is not obtained. Design effect calculates this variability compared with SRS. Design effect is a number. Here, I am not describing how to calculate this. To achieve same level of accuracy as in SRS, no of samples in SRS is to be multiplied by this design effect derived from other sampling technique. If sample size using SRS is 150 and design effect such as in cluster sampling is 3, then actual sample required is 450.

Chapter 15: Sample Size Calculation

Section 1: Concept behind Sample Size Calculation

Sample size determination is done in two situations – one is for estimation and other is for hypothesis testing. Estimation of sample size is done in cross sectional/descriptive/survey research whereas hypothesis testing is done in analytical study.

Things to Consider during Sample Size Calculation
- SD or proportion of the outcome variable being studied
- Z_α value for desired level of significance
- State one or two tailed hypothesis
- Difference we want to detect precision/margin of error
- Z_β value for desired power of the study applicable for hypothesis testing in analytical study

Adjustments during Sample Size Calculation
- Population size –finite/infinite
- Method of sampling – SRS/other method of sampling
- Unequal group size
- Expected response rate
- Number of confounding variables

Formula for Sample Size Calculation

Basic formula for sample size calculation is based on calculation of standard normal deviate Z. We know Z = Observed Difference (d)/ (SEM)

Now SEM = SD/√n. We may write $Z\alpha = d/(\frac{SD}{\sqrt{n}})$

So, √n = Zα * SD/d. Therefore $n = \frac{Z_\alpha^2 \times SD^2}{d^2}$. It is easy to remember these formulae when we calculate sample size for hypothesis testing, Z_α is replaced by ($Z_\alpha + Z_\beta$). We calculate sample size for Estimation and Hypothesis testing, method of calculation differs.

Section 2: Sample Size Calculation

Sample Size for Estimation

Scenario 1: Sample size for estimating a mean

Formula $n = \frac{z_\alpha^2 \sigma^2}{d^2}$ (Z_α is 1.96 at 5% level of significance, 2.58 at 1% level of significance and is two tailed), d = Allowable error

Problem 1: I want to estimate sample size for mean fasting blood glucose level in a community at 95% confidence limit and estimate should lie within 5mg% of true value on either side, population SD being 12mg%.

Putting all the values in formula, we get $n = \frac{(1.96)^2 \times (12)^2}{(5)^2}$. Which means I need to have at least 22 subjects in order to get an estimate of the mean fasting glucose level and the estimate that I get, 95 % of the time will be within 5 units this side or that side of the true population mean of glucose level in that community.

Problem 2: Estimate sample size for mean fasting blood glucose level in a community at 95% CI and allowable error 2.5mg% where mean fasting sugar 110mg%, population SD 12mg%.

Here $d = 2.5\% \; of \; 110 = 2.75$. So, $n = \frac{(1.96)^2 \times (12)^2}{(2.75)^2} = 73$

Scenario 2: Sample size for estimating proportion

$n = \frac{z_\alpha^2 pq}{d^2}$ (p=Proportion of the characteristic, $q = 1 - p$)

Problem 3: I want to estimate sample size to obtain an estimate of death rate due to ARI in a community 95% confidence limit and 20% allowable error, previous studies death rate due to ARI is 3%.

Here, $p = 0.03, q = 1 - 0.3 = 0.97$
and $d = 20\% \; of \; 0.03 = 0.006$.

Putting all these value in the formula, we get $n = \frac{1.96^2 \times (0.03) \times (0.97)}{0.006^2}$

Two points to note here, above two formulae are based on simple random sampling and population is finite. So, adjustment needed.

Finite population- First calculate sample size from infinite population. Now if finite population is N, then Required sample size = $\frac{n}{\left(1 + \frac{n}{N}\right)}$

If the method of sampling is other than SRS, then design effect should be calculated which the ratio of standard error is using the sample design to the standard error when SRS is used. Estimated sample size is multiplied by design effect to have actual sample size.

Scenario 3: Sample size for diagnostic test study

Step 1: Calculate R

where $R = \dfrac{\text{Sensitivity} \times (1-\text{Sensitivity})}{(\text{Acceptable deviation of expected sensitivity})^2}$

Step 2: $n = \dfrac{R}{\text{Prevalence of the disease}}$ (Each subject being evaluated with both diagnostic test and gold standard)

Problem 4: Suppose we are validating a test kit X for typhoid fever, rough estimate of sensitivity being 88% and acceptable deviation 4% on either side (84% to 92%). So, $R = \dfrac{(0.88) \times (1-0.88)}{(0.04)^2} = 66$.

Now if the prevalence of typhoid 3%, $n = \dfrac{66}{0.03} = 2200$

Sample Size for Hypothesis Testing

Scenario 1: Sample size for testing population mean with hypothesized mean (one sample t test)

$n = \dfrac{(Z_\alpha + Z_\beta)^2 \sigma^2}{(\mu_1 - \mu_2)^2}$ (μ_1 and μ_0 are population and hypothesized mean)

Problem 5: What is the sample size required to test the difference of a new antihypertensive drug in reduction of BP in compared with a standard drug whose mean reduction is 10 mmHg. Assuming mean and SD of the test drug 20 and 12 (from previous studies).

This is two tailed test. Putting all those values, we get $n = \dfrac{(1.96+0.84)^2 \times (12)^2}{(20-10)^2} = 12$

Scenario 2: Sample size calculation for hypothesis testing for diff between two means

Formula $n = \dfrac{(Z_\alpha + Z_\beta)^2 \times (\sigma_1^2 + \sigma_2^2)}{d^2}$ where Z_β value is for power of the study, usually 80% power is accepted. If σ_1 and σ_2 are same and equal to σ, $n = 2 \times \dfrac{(Z_\alpha + Z_\beta)^2 \times \sigma^2}{d^2}$

Problem 6: We want to study the effect of a new antihypertensive drug and comparing with standard drug in the market at 95% confidence limit.

Experimental group is given new drug and control group received standard drug. Standard deviation from previous study 10mmHg, we expect difference in BP after treatment is 8 mm Hg. power of the study 80%, hence $Z_\beta = 0.84$

It is a two tailed test. So, $n = 2 \times \dfrac{(Z_\alpha+Z_\beta)^2 \times \sigma^2}{d^2} = 2 \times \dfrac{(1.96+0.84)^2 \times (10)^2}{(8)^2}$.

We should recruit 25 subjects in experimental gr and 25 subjects in control group.

Scenario 3: Testing proportion with fixed value- binary outcome

Formula $n = \dfrac{(Z_\alpha\sqrt{p_0 q_0} + Z_\beta\sqrt{p_1 q_1})^2}{(p_1-p_0)^2}$

Scenario 4: Sample size calculation for hypothesis testing for diff between two Proportions

$n = \dfrac{(Z_\alpha+Z_\beta)^2 \times (p_0 q_0 + p_1 q_1)}{(p_1-p_0)^2}$. If response of one group known,

$n = \dfrac{(Z_\alpha+Z_\beta)^2 \times 2pq}{(\text{Difference in response desired})^2}$

Problem 7: Investigator wants to calculate the sample size of each group where he compares the success rate of new drug (80%) with standard drug (success rate 68%), consider 80% power and at 95% confidence limit, it is one tail so $Z_\alpha = 1.645$

Here $p_0 = 0.68, q_0 = 0.32, p_1 = 0.8, q_1 = 0.2$

Putting all these values in the formula $n = \dfrac{(Z_\alpha+Z_\beta)^2 \times (p_0 q_0 + p_1 q_1)}{(p_1-p_0)^2}$, we get

$n = \dfrac{(1.64+0.84)^2 \times [(0.68*0.32)+(0.8*0.2)]}{(0.80-0.68)^2} = 161$.

So, for each group, 161 subjects are required for comparison.

Problem 8: Investigator wants to calculate the sample size of each group where he compares the success rate of new drug with standard drug (success rate 80%), desired difference in response rate (absolute value) is 10%, consider 80% power and at 95% confidence limit, it is two tailed, so $Z_\alpha = 1.96$

Here $n = \dfrac{(Z_\alpha+Z_\beta)^2 \times 2pq}{(Difference\ in\ Response\ Desired)^2}$.

Putting all the values, $n = \dfrac{2 \times (1.96+0.84)^2 \times (0.8*0.2)}{(0.1)^2} = 251$ subjects /group.

Sometimes in sample size calculation, measures of effect size are specified. This effect size measure in case control study is odds ratio and in cohort study it is relative risk. In this situation, formula for testing the difference between two proportions is modified. Remember, outcome here measured is binary in nature.

In prospective (cohort /clinical trial) study:

P_O = Proportion of subjects without exposure at risk of developing disease and relative risk are to be specified (other than alpha and power) before calculation.

Similarly, in case control study:

P_O = Proportion of subjects without outcome who are likely to have exposure and odds ratio are to be specified (other than alpha and power) before calculation. Once OR/RR and P_O are given, we can calculate P_1 in the following way:

In prospective study: $P_1 = \dfrac{P_0 \times RR}{[1 + P_0(RR-1)]}$

In case control study, $P_1 = \dfrac{P_0 \times OR}{[1 + P_0(OR-1)]}$. Then we can find out value of p and q which is as follows: $p = \dfrac{P_0 + P_1}{2}, q = 1 - p$

We calculate sample size with the formula: $n = \dfrac{(Z_\alpha + Z_\beta)^2 \times pq}{(p_1 - p_0)^2}$

Scenario 5: Paired t test (before and after test, continuous outcome)

Formula $n = \dfrac{(Z_\alpha + Z_\beta)^2 \times \sigma^2}{d^2}$ where σ is the standard deviation of the variable under study and d is difference desired after treatment

Problem 9: A new lipid lowering agent is being tested for its hypolipidemic effect using same subjects (before and after) to detect a difference of 10 mmHg of BP. Standard deviation of the variable (BP) from pilot study being 12mm Hg. What sample size is required at 95% confidence limit with 80% power of study?

Investigator here using the same subjects as his control, paired observation is taken into account. Putting all these value in the formula, we get $n = \dfrac{(1.96+0.84)^2 \times (12)^2}{(10)^2} = 12$

So, 12 subjects will be given lipid lowering agent after taking blood for initial lipid level (say serum cholesterol) and after a specific time period (say 12 weeks), again they will be tested for lipid level. Finally, to mention here that 10% extra subjects to be included for non-responders, same principle applies when 10% extra added per confounding variable. Correction or adjustment is necessary for unequal group size.

When there are multiple outcome variables, sample size for each to be calculated and that maximum value is to be considered for study. There are many types of study design and analysis method. Examples discussed above are easy to calculate manually. In other cases, we take the help of software. Free software available are OpenEpi, G Power. We can easily calculate sample size for ANOVA, regression analysis.

Sample Size in Animal Study

Most preferred method of calculating sample size is the same as which is used for hypothesis testing. Sometimes, information necessary for calculation are not available, in that condition, we use 'Resource Equation Method'.

In this method, a value E is calculated based on decided sample size where E = Total number of animals − number of groups. For optimal sample size, E value should lie between 10 to 20. More animals to be added if it is <10 and number of animals should be reduced if E value is > 20.

Problem 10: We want to test the effect of hypolipidemic drugs on serum cholesterol level in 5 groups of rats. One group is control; other groups receive 4 different drugs. What is the minimum number of rats / group?

If we take 5 groups of animals, then keep E value between 10 to 20 (use 'Resource Equation Method'). Suppose we are taking E value of 20, then $20 = X - 5$. Thus, X = Total number of animals = 25

As a result, Number of animals in each group = $\frac{25}{5} = 5$

Chapter 16: Systematic Review

Section 1: Systematic Review and Metanalysis

Introduction

"Systematic review" refers to a process of collecting, evaluating, and synthesizing all available evidence, while the term "meta-analysis" refers to the statistical technique involved in extracting and combining data to produce a summary result. The researchers use an organized method of locating, assembling, and evaluating a body of literature on a particular topic using a set of specific criteria. To improve scientific writing, standard reporting format is there such as PRISMA (Preferred Reporting Items in Systematic review and Meta analysis) for RCTs and Meta-analysis of observational studies in epidemiology (MOOSE) for observational data. A systematic review can be either quantitative or qualitative. Before going for systematic review, it is desirable to register at PROSPERO at protocol stage to avoid any bias.

Skill Development

Step 1: Formulate a question
Step 2: Develop protocol
Step 3: Review literature -electronic scientific database, the popular ones are PUBMED, MEDLINE, and EMBASE
Step 4: Select studies and assess study quality
Step 5: Calculate effect size based on outcome measures
Binary - Odds Ratio/Risk Ratio
Continuous- standardized difference in means
Time to event - Hazard Ratio
Step 6: Combining results– before combining each result, homogeneity from the graph usually forest plot is assessed. Definitive test for assessing heterogeneity Mantel-Haenszel test. Finally, common estimate and CI from each study is calculated.
Step 7: Interpret results–Forest plot (Image 1) gives graphical representation of each study result and also overall estimate. In forest plot different information is in different column: Study ID, intervention

and control group, a vertical line representing a line of effect, each study results (includes effect size and CI) and diamond in last row representing Overall Estimate. Horizontal lines represent each study results with CI and square in it being effect size.

Step 8: Subgroup and sensitivity analysis in last step

Construction of Forest Plot in Excel (Table 1)

Table 1: Dataset of Forest Plot

Study ID	Effect Size	LCL	Negative Error Bar	UCL	Positive Error Bar	Position
Study 1						
Study 2						
Study 3						
Study 4						
Study 5						
Study 6						

Advantages of Systematic Review
- ❖ Chances of bias less
- ❖ Reliable and accurate conclusions
- ❖ Quickly dissemination of information
- ❖ Can generalize our search results
- ❖ Generates new hypotheses
- ❖ Increases precision

Limitation of Systematic Review
- ❖ Location and selection of studies
- ❖ Heterogeneity
- ❖ Absence of important outcomes
- ❖ Inappropriate subgroup analyses
- ❖ Duplication of publication
- ❖ Publication bias

Biostatistics in Health Research

Image 1: Forest Plot

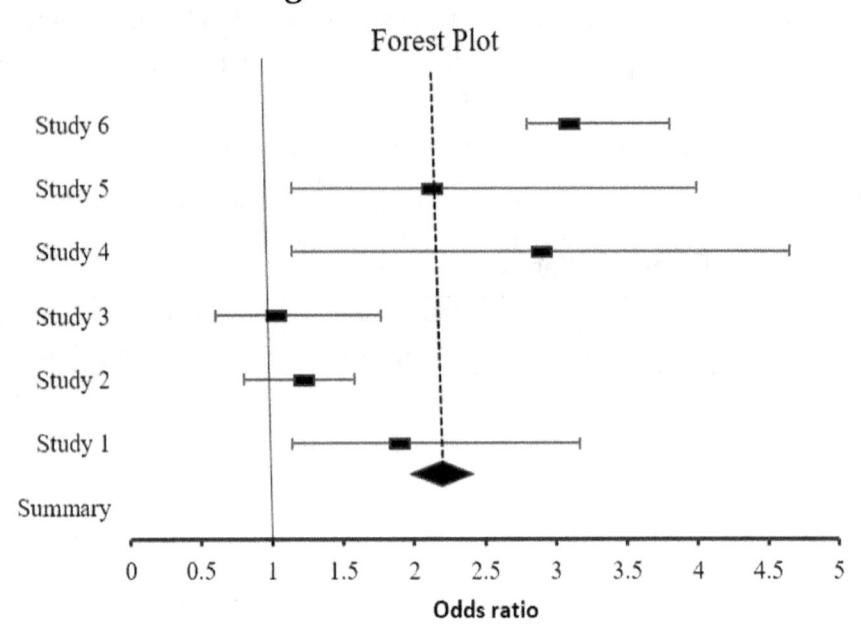

Biostatistics in Health Research

Section 2: FAQ on Systematic Review

1. Prepare a flow chart for conducting systematic review
2. What are the objectives of Systematic review?
   It contributes to evidence-based practice
   Large amount of information summarized in an easy comprehensive form to help busy clinician (Reliable basis for decision making)
3. How many researchers are required for systematic review?
   Three (two independent reviewers and one arbitrator to solve any conflict between reviewers)
4. Write down two disadvantages of Systematic review.
   - Introduction of bias -Selection bias, publication bias
   - Selective outcome reporting
5. Name some database from where we retrieve data for systematic review. (Google Scholar, PubMed, Cochrane)
6. Write differences between Narrative and systematic review.
7. Write difference between systematic review and meta-analysis?
   Meta-analysis is statistical counterpart of systematic review.
8. What is the minimum number of studies required for systematic review?
9. What is the minimum number of study in meta-analysis?
   Minimum of two with similar results that can be combined.
10. Write down purposes of meta-analysis.
    - Estimation of treatment effect
    - Amount of variability detection
    - Magnitude of risk(harm/benefit)
11. What are the different types of analysis done in meta-analysis?
12. Name two software used in Systematic reviews.
    Rayyan, COVIDENCE, SYSREV
13. Name two software used in meta-analysis.
    RevMan, MS-EXCEL, STATA, R software (Metafor), Python
14. What is average time taken to do a systematic review?
    Six to 18months
15. Name some organizations that work on syntheses of evidence in the form of systematic reviews
    Equator Network, JBI Collaboration, Cochrane Collaboration and Campbell Collaboration.
16. Why not simple average of summary statistic of each study?

Simple averaging gives equal weight to each study whereas results of some studies are closer to the actual value or true value. So, weight should reflect actual study strength.

17. Write difference between systematic and systematized review?
Exhaustive comprehensive searching and quality assessment is usually minimal in systematized review.
What is the first step in systematic review? (Research question)

18. What does PICO(ST) stand for?
P-Population/problem, I- Intervention, C-comparator/placebo, O-outcome/effect, S-Study design, T-time frame.

19. Classify different type research questions for systematic review?
Incidence, prevalence, prognosis, diagnostic accuracy etc.

20. How to write eligibility criteria of studies for systematic review?
Should match with PICO(ST)

21. What is Prisma P and PROSPERO?
Prisma P-Preferred Reporting Items for Systematic review and Meta-Analysis Protocols, PROSPERO-Prospective Register of Systematic Reviews

22. What is Heterogeneity? Write sources of it. Describe graphical and statistical method of identification of Heterogeneity?

23. What is meta regression, subgroup analysis and sensitivity analysis? How these different techniques explore heterogeneity?

24. What will you do if significant heterogeneity?

25. What is Forest plot?

26. Role of Funnel plot in detecting bias-Discuss.

27. Write different tools used for systematic review and specify purpose for each of them. (reference to Cochrane database search)

28. Discuss plagiarism aspect while performing systematic review.

29. Arrange the following in correct sequence: PROSPERO registration, Protocol writing (PRISMA P), Searching literature.
Protocol writing as per PRISMA P format then Registration at PROSPERO then Searching literature

Section 3: Systematic Review Process (Flow Chart)

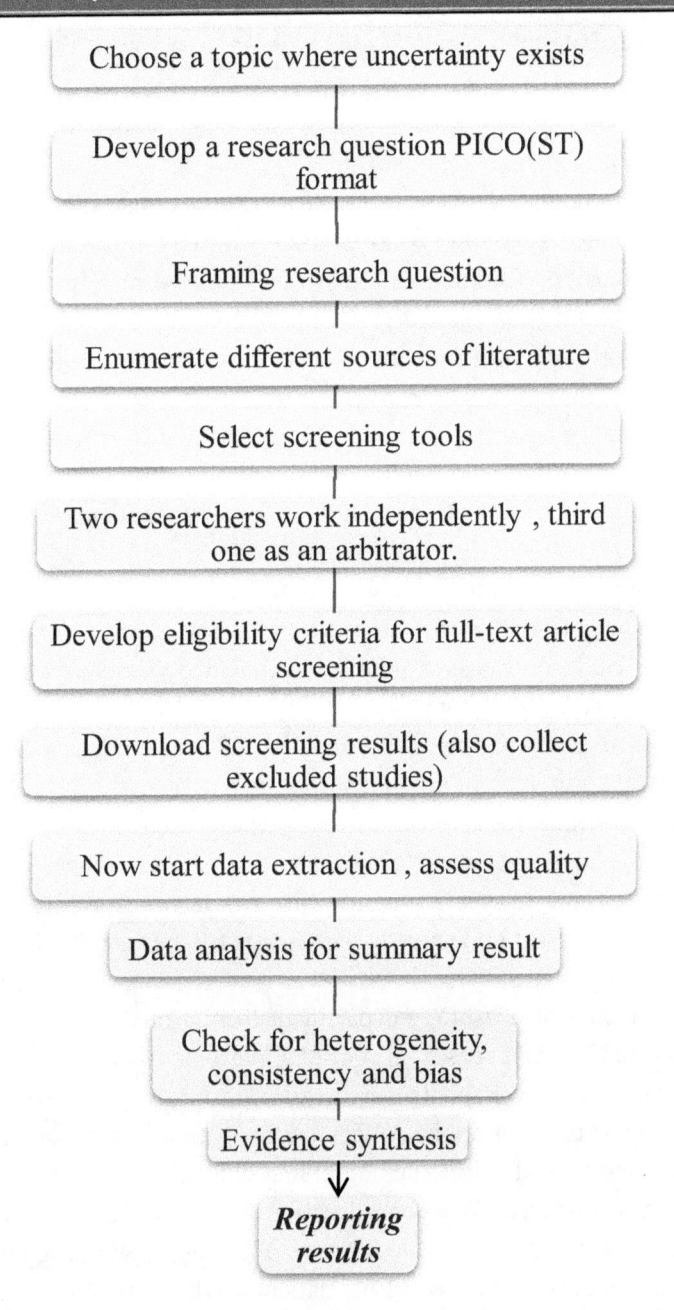

- Choose a topic where uncertainty exists
- Develop a research question PICO(ST) format
- Framing research question
- Enumerate different sources of literature
- Select screening tools
- Two researchers work independently, third one as an arbitrator.
- Develop eligibility criteria for full-text article screening
- Download screening results (also collect excluded studies)
- Now start data extraction, assess quality
- Data analysis for summary result
- Check for heterogeneity, consistency and bias
- Evidence synthesis
- ***Reporting results***

Chapter 17: Assessments

Section 1: Type of Study

1. Investigator wants to know the prevalence of leprosy in the district X during 1st Jan 2021 to 31st Dec 2021 and collecting information. *(Descriptive Cross sectional)*
2. Epidemiologist is doing community survey and measuring BP of individuals aged 40 years and above to estimate prevalence of hypertension (defined as Systolic BP>140mmHg or Diastolic BP>90mmHg). *(Descriptive Cross sectional)*
3. Antibiotic prescription pattern in NICU of Burdwan Medical College and Hospital in WB. *(Descriptive Cross sectional)*
4. We want to see trend of Covid -19 in coming year (Month wise cases). *(Descriptive longitudinal)*
5. Behaviour of relatives with Covid-19 patients. *(Descriptive longitudinal)*
6. Epidemiologist went to a village and tried to find causes of recent outbreak of AGE in the community. He is recording information in texts. He also discussed with some educated groups of people in that area. *(Qualitative research)*
7. Head of the department of Medicine of a hospital is reporting in a journal a rare case of blood disorder. *(Case report)*
8. To determine the association between breast cancer and per capita dietary fat intake, data for prevalence of breast cancer from cancer registry and of per capita dietary fat intake from national level information was collected for 6 countries for the year 2014. *(Ecological or correlation study)*
9. A clinician of neurology department from a medical college in India reported 12 rare cases of familial periodic paralysis in a famous research article. Patients were available from August 2020 to October 2020 and the neurologist collected information from those patients. He described details of the demographic, clinical, and laboratory features of those rare case. What best describes this study design? *(Case series)*
10. To determine the associated factors of antipsychotic drug compliance, a psychiatrist selected 152 patients with MDD who were on antipsychotic drug therapy in a tertiary care hospital. He collected the details on the personal background of the subjects and also took history of medications in past one month. Drug compliant group and the non-

compliant group were compared to identify associated risk factors. What best describes the design? *(Analytical cross sectional)*

11. Using cancer registry of a hospital, a researcher collected data on chemical exposure of workers and bladder carcinoma on patients admitted between 1990 and 2005. Patients were classified as exposed who had history of working in dye industry and others as unexposed. He then compared the frequency of bladder carcinoma among the exposed and the unexposed. *(Retrospective cohort)*

12. A researcher is determining association between smoking and carcinoma stomach. He conducted the study involving large geographical region. 150 patients of lung cancer selected, 300 subjects without chosen as control. Both cases and control were comparable at the base level with respect to demographic variables. They were asked about their smoking habits. Presence of smoking habit is a risk factor. Now the association between lung cancer and smoking was determined. *(Case control study)*

13. A physiologist decided to conduct a study to investigate association between exercise and coronary heart disease. He defined exercise as 45 min continuous walking/jogging or cycling in a day for 5 days in a week. Coronary heart disease is outcome here and specified as ST segment changes. Subjects included 30-50years. He selected 200 subjects in one group and they are not doing exercise and another group of 200 subjects are taking exercises. Both groups were screened for coronary artery disease before start of the study and subjects having ST segment changes were excluded from the study. Now both groups are followed up over a period of 10 years. Then each individual in both groups were screened for ECG changes. Association between ECG changes and exercise is determined.
Which test? –*Chi-square test*
What type of study design? - *Prospective cohort study*
What is the measure of association? -*Relative risk*

14. A medical college of West Bengal will conduct a study to assess the efficacy of a Covishield vaccine for the prevention of Covid 19 in children aged 2-12years. Randomization will be done. Efficacy of Covishield will be assessed 15 days after completion of 2nd dose to 9months and compared with non-vaccinated children. Diagnosis of Covid19 will be by RTPCR. *(Prophylactic RCT/Preventive trial)*

15. Which is the best method to ensure that the treatment and control arms in a clinical trial are identical with respect to confounders at the start of study? *(Randomization)*
16. Researcher from surgery department compared the wound healing time between conventional suturing technique and stapling technique for closure of surgical site incision. Patients were unaware about the treatment assignment. *(Single blind RCT)*
17. Researcher from surgery department compared the wound healing time between conventional suturing technique and stapling technique for closure of surgical site incision. Patients and the researcher were aware about the treatment assignment. *(Open label RCT)*
18. An epidemiologist visits a remote tribal area, discussed with them about myths and taboos of snake bite cases. *(Qualitative research)*
19. An epidemiologist visits a remote tribal area and discussed with them about myths and taboos of snake bite cases. He also estimates prevalence of snake bite cases in that area to plan health care services. *(Mixed study design)*
20. An investigator decided to estimate the prevalence of grade1 hypertension among middle aged men with BMI >22 in Purba Burdwan. But he recruited subjects from Medicine OPD of Burdwan Medical College &Hospital. Identify Target Population and Accessible Population here.

Section 2: Type of Analysis

1. An existing antihypertensive drug reduces systolic BP on an average of 15 mmHg. A company claims that a new drug X is equally effective and also safe. Researcher recruited 40 patients with hypertension and drug administered. After 12 days of therapy their BP recorded compared with mean BP reduction of 15mmHg by standard drug. (One Sample t Test)
2. A new vaccine against Covid-19 has been launched and the manufacturer claims that it is effective in 85% of cases. In order to verify claim, we selected 400 vaccinated individuals after 9 months of vaccination in our medical college setting. We found that 280 individuals were protected. We want to test whether observed efficacy is significantly different what the company claims. (One Sample Test of Proportion)
3. Study to find median hospital stay following infant diarrhoea when probiotic is added is statistically different from 3 days. Data collected from 50 patients with probiotics. (One Sample Median test)
4. An investigator wants to study whether there is any difference in systolic BP between two groups of patients, each group consist of 10 individuals. (Independent t Test)
5. Testing efficacy of a new antihypertensive drug, Researcher recruited 15 patients of either sex and recorded their initial BP and again after 12 days of therapy. (Paired t Test)
6. To test whether a new and Covishield vaccine is preventing Covid19, investigator recruited vaccinated subjects who completed 2 doses of the vaccine and also a second group of subjects who have not taken vaccine. Both groups will be followed up for 9 months for any symptoms of the disease. Confirmation of the disease will be by RTPCR. Data collected includes number of subjects developed the disease in both the groups. (Chi-Square Test of Independence)
7. In a study, an Investigator recruited ninety patients of grade I hypertension and tested three drugs-Drug X, Drug Y and Drug Z. They received Drug for 45 days, with a gap of 15 days. At the end of 45 days BP recorded in each time. How to test the efficacy of these three drugs? (One-way Repeated Measure ANOVA)
8. In a cross-sectional survey, an epidemiologist interviewed 400 persons of ages between 30-70 years about their social class and recorded their

BP. He divided into three age groups: upper class, middle class and lower class. BP recording will classify them as normotensive and hypertensive. Test whether social class has an influence on BP? (Chi-Square Test for Trend)

9. Suppose, an awareness program of about health hazards of smoking was conducted among 100 adult participants. Some of the participants were smokers and some of them were non-smokers. After the program, we again counted number of smokers and non-smokers, in addition to that we counted participants who changed their habit (from smoker to non-smoker, from non-smoker to smoker). Does the awareness program have significant impact on habit. (Mc Nemar Test)

10. Investigator selected 50 patients in each group (based on grades of hypertension). On ECG, ischaemic changes found in 5,8, 12 patients in grade I, grade II, grade III hypertension patients. Researcher wants to know whether this difference in ischemic changes is related with grades of hypertension or due to chance? (Chi-square Test for Goodness of Fit)

11. In medicine OPD of our Medical College &Hospital, 60 patients with hypertension were included in the study to find whether BMI, Age and Serum Cholesterol level can influence BP of an individual. (Multiple Linear Regression)

12. Clinician in a Covid 19 ward, collected blood samples to measure viral load from 300 patients. He suspected that viral load may predict respiratory distress requiring ventilation. He prepared range of cut-off values of viral load and wants to know the useful cut-off value which has more likelihood of developing severe respiratory symptoms. (ROC Curve).

13. A psychiatrist recruited 120 patients of major depressive disorder and divided them randomly into four groups. His interest is to find whether type of therapy (Psychodynamic and CBT) and Drug (here Escitalopram and MAO inhibitor) have impact (interaction) on lowering depression score (as per Beck Depression Inventory). He divided groups as follows: Escitalopram with CBT (Group I), Escitalopram with Psychodynamic therapy (Group II), MAO inhibitor with CBT (Group III) and MAO inhibitor with Psychodynamic therapy (Group IV). How to analyse response.

Bibliography

1. Bhalwar R. Textbook of Public Health and Community Medicine. 1st edition. Dept. of Community Medicine, AFMC Pune in collaboration with WHO, India Office, New Delhi. 2009
2. Multifaculty from ICMR-National Institute of Epidemiology (ICMR-NIE). Basic course in Biomedical Research-Cycle 3. National Programme on Technology Enhanced Learning. 2020. Available: https://onlinecourses.nptel.ac.in/noc20_md03/preview
3. Field A. Discovering statistics using SPSS. 3rd Edition. SAGE Publications Ltd.2009.
4. Health Research Methodology: A Guide for Training in Research Methods. 2nd Edition. World Health Organization, Regional Office for the Western Pacific, Manila. 2001
5. Hulley SB, Cummings SR, Browner WS, Grady DG, Newman TB. Designing Clinical Research. 4th Edition. Lippincott Williams & Wilkins, a Wolters Kluwer business. 2013.
6. Park K. Park's Textbook of Preventive and Social Medicine. 26th Edition. Banarsidas Bhanot Publishers; 2021.
7. Biostatistics and Design of experiments - Course [Internet]. [cited 2023 Jul 7]. Available: https://onlinecourses.nptel.ac.in/noc20_bt11/preview
8. Manikandan S. Data transformation. J Pharmacol Pharmacother. 2010;1(2):126–7.
9. Parikh MN, Hazra A, Mukherjee J, Gogtay N. Research Methodology Simplified: Every Clinician a Researcher. 1st ed. New Delhi: Jaypee Brothers Medical Publishers; 2010.
10. Wasserstein RL, Lazar NA. The ASA statement on p-values: context, process, and purpose.
11. Burt T, Young G, Lee W, Kusuhara H, Langer O, Rowland M, Sugiyama Y. Phase 0/microdosing approaches: time for mainstream application in drug development? Nature Reviews Drug Discovery. 2020 Nov; 19(11):801-18.
12. Fromer MJ.FDA introduces new phase 0 for clinical trials:some enthusiastic, some skeptical. Oncology Times.2006 Aug10; 28(15):18-9.
13. In J. Introduction of a pilot study. Korean J Anesthesiol. 2017; 70(6):601-5.
14. Hassan ZA, Schattner P, Mazza D. Doing A Pilot Study: Why Is It Essential? Malays Fam Physician. 2006; 1(2-3):70-3.
15. Stewart PW. Small or pilot study, GCRC protocols which propose "pilot studies". Cincinnati Children's Hospital Medical Center
16. Lim CY, In J. Randomization in clinical studies. Korean J Anesthesiol. 2019 Apr 1;72(3):221–32.

17. Research C for DE and. Surrogate Endpoint Resources for Drug and Biologic Development. FDA [Internet]. 2021 Jan 29 [cited 2023 Jul 6]; Available from: https://www.fda.gov/drugs/development-resources/surrogate-endpoint-resources-drug-and-biologic-development
18. Petrie A, Sabin C. Medical statistics at a glance. Oxford ; Malden, MA: Blackwell Science; 2000. 138 p
19. How to perform a Mixed ANOVA in SPSS Statistics | Laerd Statistics [Internet]. [cited 2023 Jul 7]. Available from: https://statistics.laerd.com/spss-tutorials/mixed-ANOVA-using-spss-statistics.php
20. How to perform a two-way repeated measures ANOVA in SPSS Statistics | Laerd Statistics [Internet]. [cited 2023 Jul 7]. Available from: https://statistics.laerd.com/spss-tutorials/two-way-repeated-measures-ANOVA-using-spss-statistics.php
21. Nonparametric Tests [Internet]. [cited 2023 Jul 7]. Available from: https://sphweb.bumc.bu.edu/otlt/mph modules/bs/bs704_nonparametric/bs704_nonparametric_print.html
22. Field-Fote E [Edee. Mediators and Moderators, Confounders and Covariates: Exploring the Variables That Illuminate or Obscure the "Active Ingredients" in Neurorehabilitation. J Neurol Phys Ther. 2019 Apr;43(2):83.
23. Mahajan BK. Methods in biostatistics. Jaypee Brothers Publishers; 2002.
24. Latin_Square_(revised).pdf [Internet]. [cited 2023 Jul 7]. Available: https://www.ndsu.edu/faculty/horsley/Latin_Square_(revised).pdf
25. sec3c.pdf [Internet]. [cited 2023 Jul 7]. Available from: https://math.montana.edu/jobo/st541/sec3c.pdf
26. Probit Regression | Stata Data Analysis Examples [Internet]. [cited 2023 Jul 6]. Available from: https://stats.oarc.ucla.edu/stata/dae/probit-regression/
27. Daines R. LibGuides: Statistics Resources: Binomial Logistic Regression [Internet]. [cited 2023 Jul 6]. Available from: https://resources.nu.edu/statsresources/Binomiallogistic
28. How to perform a Binomial Logistic Regression in SPSS Statistics | Laerd Statistics [Internet]. [cited 2023 Jul 6]. Available from: https://statistics.laerd.com/spss-tutorials/binomial-logistic-regression-using-spss-statistics.php
29. Ghosh MN. Fundamentals of Experimental Pharmacology. 7th ed. Kolkata: Hilton & Company; 2019.
30. Kulkarni SK. Hand Book of Experimental Pharmacology, Vallabh Prakashan, Delhi, 3rd Rev.

31. Pannucci CJ, Wilkins EG. Identifying and Avoiding Bias in Research. Plast Reconstr Surg. 2010 Aug;126(2):619–25.
32. Lise Lotte Gluud, Bias in Clinical Intervention Research, American Journal of Epidemiology, Volume 163, Issue 6, 15 March 2006, Pages 493–501, https://doi.org/10.1093/aje/kwj069
33. Giavarina D. Understanding Bland Altman analysis. Biochem Medica. 2015 Jun 5;25(2):141–51.
34. Ranganathan P, Pramesh CS, Aggarwal R. Common pitfalls in statistical analysis: Measures of agreement. Perspect Clin Res. 2017;8(4):187–91.
35. Kaplan-Meier method in SPSS Statistics | Laerd Statistics [Internet]. [cited 2023 Jul 6]. Available from: https://statistics.laerd.com/spss-tutorials/kaplan-meier-using-spss-statistics.php
36. Festing MF. Design and statistical methods in studies using animal models of development. ILAR J. 2006; 47:5–14.
37. Arifin WN, Zahiruddin WM. Sample Size Calculation in Animal Studies Using Resource Equation Approach. Malays J Med Sci MJMS. 2017 Oct;24(5):101–5.
38. Gopalakrishnan S, Ganeshkumar P. Systematic reviews and meta-analysis: understanding the best evidence in primary healthcare. Journal of family medicine and primary care. 2013 Jan; 2(1):9.
39. Ahn E, Kang H. Introduction to systematic review and meta-analysis. Korean J Anesthesiol. 2018; 71(2):103-112. doi:10.4097/kjae.2018.71.2.103
40. PubMed tutorials: https://learn.nlm.nih.gov/documentation/training-packets/T0042010P/
41. Literature search demo_Lecture handout.pdf [Internet]. Google Docs. [cited 2023 Jan 21]. Available from: https://drive.google.com/file/d/1GbxRSaFWXt9EgMCEziTXx_d62vpMX1zR/view?usp=sharing&usp=embed_facebook
42. NIeCer 104: Introduction to Systematic Reviews for Dental Health Professionals - Course [Internet]. [cited 2023 Feb 2]. Available from: https://onlinecourses.swayam2.ac.in/aic21_ge26/preview.

INDEX

A
Accessible Population 162
Accuracy 147
Addition Rule 2
Adjusted R^2 130
Allocation Concealment 49
Alpha Error 28
Alternate Hypothesis 26
Ambispective Cohort 45
Area Sampling 169
Arithmetic Mean 6
Ascertainment 141
Assessment Bias 141

B
Berkson's Bias 140
Beta Error 28
Between-Groups SS 84
Between-Subjects Variable 100
Bias Due to Nonresponse 140
Binomial Distribution 23
Blinding 49
Box and Whisker Plot 16

C
Carry Over Effect 124
Case Control Study 41
Censoring 158
Census 161
CFR 59
Chance 33
Clinical Trial 46
Cluster Sampling 166
Cohen's d 33
Cohort Study 43
Confidence Interval 30
Confidence Interval of Odds Ratio 61
Confidence Level 30
Confidence Limit 31
Confounder 133
Confounding Bias 142
Confounding Variable 56
Construct Validity 145
Content Analysis 40
Content Validity 144
Content Validity Index 144
Control Group 49
Control of Confounding 56
Covariate 133
Covariates 97
Cox & Snell R^2 136
Cox Regression 159
Criterion Validity 145
Cronbach's Alpha (A) 146
Cross Over Design 119

Cross Sectional Study 45
Cumulative Incidence 59
CV 11
CVI 144

D
Data 1
Degree Of Freedom 76
Dependent Events 2
Dependent Variable 107
Descriptive Statistics 65
Design Effect 169
Discriminant Validity 145

E
Ecological Study 41
Effect Size 33
Error 137
Error Term 137
External Validity 144

F
F Statistic 34
F Test 70
F Value 82
Face Validity 144
FGD 40
Fixed-Effects Model(ANOVA) 88
Focus Group Discussions 40
Forest Plot 176
Fractional Factorial Design 124
Full Factorial Design 123

G
Geometric Mean 6
Grounded Theory 40

H
Harmonic Mean 6
Histogram 17
Homoscedasticity 132
Hosmer-Lemeshow Test 136
Hypothesis Testing 26

I
Incidence 59
Incidence Density 59
Incidence Rate 59
Independent Events 2
Independent Variable 107
In-Depth (Individual) Interviews 39
Inferential Statistics 65
Information Bias 141
Inter Quartile Range 7
Interaction Effect 86
Interaction Plot 87
Internal Consistency 145
Inter-Observer Reliability 146

INDEX

Interval Scale 5
K
Kaplan-Meier Method 158
KM Plot 158
Kurtosis 69
L
Latin Square Design 121
Laws of Probability 2
Ld50 138
Levene's Test 69, 70
Log Linear Regression 113
Log Rank Test 159
Logarithm 3
Logit Function 135
Lr(-) 151
Lr(+) 151
M
Mann Whitney Test 118
MANOVA 107
Mc Nemar Test 113
Median 6
Mediator 132
Mixed-Effects Model(ANOVA) 88
Mode 6
Model 1
Moderators 133
MOOSE 176
Multicollinearity 132
Multiplication Rule 2
Multi-Stage Sampling 167
Mutually Exclusive Events 2
N
Nagalkerke R^2 136
NNH 64
NNT 64
Non- Sampling Error 161
Normal Distribution 21
NPV 149
Null Hypothesis 26
O
Odds 61
Odds Ratio 61
OFAT 107, 123
Ogives 14
One Tailed Test 29
Outlier 71
P
Partial Correlation 128
Participant Observations 40
Period Prevalence 59
Phi and Cramer's V 109
Pilot Study 50
Point Prevalence 59
Poisson Distribution 22
Poisson Regression 134
Population 1
Power of Study 30
PPS 165
PPV 149
Precision 147
Prediction Statistics 65
Predictive Validity 145
Prevarication 141
PRISMA 176
Probability 2
Probit 139
Proportion 58
Proportional Bias 157
Prospective Cohort 44
P-Value 34
R
Random Agreement 155
Random Error 26, 33
Random-Effects Model(Anova) 88
Randomization 52
Rate 58
Ratio 58
Ratio Scale 5
Recall Bias 141
Reference Population 162
Regression Coefficient 129
Relative Risk 44
Reproducibility/ Replication 148
Residual 137
Resource Equation Method' 175
Retrospective Cohort 44
Risk 60
ROC 136
S
Sample 1
Sample Size 161
Sample Size in Animal Study 175
Sampling 161
Sampling Error 161
Sampling Fraction 161
Sampling Interval 161
Selection Bias 140
Sensitivity 148
Simple Random Sampling 163
Simple Randomization 52
Skewness 25, 69
SMART 54
Snowball Sampling 169
SPANOVA 100

INDEX

Spearman Rank Correlation Coefficient 118
Specificity 149
Sphericity 93
Spillover effect 125
SRS 163
Standard Deviation 9
Standard Error of Mean 10
Statistic 1
Statistical Table 19
Statistics 1
Stratified Sampling 166
Study Population 162
Surrogate Endpoint 50
Surveillance Bias 141
Survival 158
Survival Bias 140
Survival Function 158
Systematic Error 33
Systematic Random Sampling 164

T
Target Population 162
Test Statistics 33
Test–Re-Test Reliability 146
Third Variable 132
Two Sample Z Test For Proportions 75
Two Tailed Test 29
Type I Error 28
Type II Error 28

W
Wald Statistic 136
Welch T Test 80
Wilcoxon Signed Rank Test 117
Within-Groups SS 84
Within-Subjects Variable 100

Y
Yate's Correction 112

Z
Z Score 75
Z Test 74, 75